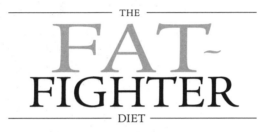

THE
FAT-
FIGHTER
DIET

THE

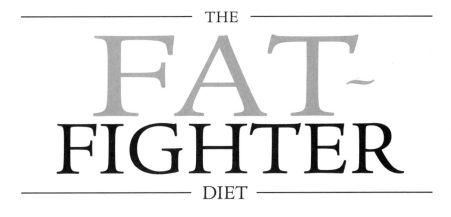

FAT-FIGHTER

DIET

BRUCE KRAHN

with holistic nutritionist Janet Hradil, R.H.N.

WILEY

John Wiley & Sons Canada, Ltd.

National Library of Canada Cataloguing in Publication Data

Krahn, Bruce
   The fat-fighter diet / Bruce Krahn.
Includes bibliographical references and index.

ISBN 978-0-470-15326-0

   1. Weight loss. 2. Reducing diets. 3. Reducing exercises.
I. Title.

RM222.2.K69 2007   613.2'5   C2007-902535-8

Production Credits
Cover design: Ian Koo
Cover photography: Top (left to right); Digital Vision, Medioimages/Photodisc, Photodisc;
   Bottom; Lorella Zanetti Photography
Interior design and typsetting: Jason Vandenberg
Interior illustrations: Imagineering Media Services Inc.
Printer: Quebecor, Taunton

John Wiley & Sons Canada, Ltd.
6045 Freemont Blvd.
Mississauga, Ontario
L5R 4J3

Printed in Canada

1 2 3 4 5 QW 11 10 09 08 07

CONTENTS

FOREWORD

As a nutritional researcher, author, and speaker, I have the privilege of interacting with people from all walks of life. I see those who are healthy and functioning at a high level as well as people who are suffering from various forms of illness and disease. Quite often I am struck by the fact that much of the sickness and health, happiness and misery that people experience are the result of the decisions and choices they make each and every day.

The Fat-Fighter Diet is about so much more than simply counting calories! In this fascinating book, Bruce combines emotional empowerment together with scientific fact while stripping away layers of half-truths and misconceptions about what it really takes to live your life in a body full of vibrant health, energy, enthusiasm, and physical fitness.

Empowering people to accept responsibility for their own happiness, health, and fitness is not always easy. However, Bruce breaks things down in an easy-to-read, easy-to-apply format that removes any guesswork. Simply decide on your goal, add a dash of determination and a sprinkle of persistence, and you will succeed!

I see Bruce as a great coach and motivator who can help you achieve your health and fitness goals. His passion and enthusiasm come through his words, encouraging you to take the actions necessary for achievement. You hold in your hands a powerful resource. I encourage you to refer to it often and reap the benefits.

I wish you abundant good health.

—Sam Graci, Author of *The Bone-Building Solution,*
Researcher and formulator of greens+

ACKNOWLEDGEMENTS

This book has been in the "works" for several years and there have been many people who have helped to bring it to fruition.

First and foremost I would like to thank my beautiful wife Janet. Her unwavering support and commitment to all of my endeavors have made all things possible for me. I do not know where I would be without her.

Heartfelt thanks to the entire team at Wiley for giving me the opportunity to have my voice heard. A special thanks to Leah Fairbank—you always make me smile—as well as Ian Koo, Elizabeth McCurdy, and Valerie Ahwee.

Thanks to the talented people at Imagineering Art.

A very special thank you to my business partner Peter Pusitz. Thanks for your support, loyalty, and always believing in the dream.

Thanks to my friend and inspiration, Sam Graci: you are a guiding light in this world. Please never stop doing what you do as the world is so much better for it.

Thanks to all of my clients to whom I am forever grateful for their ongoing support: Cathy, I know we will get there; Paul, thanks for the education; Steve, you inspire me!

Thank you to my mother and father whose love and support has given me wings on which to fly.

To my brothers Brad and Bryan—I miss you guys!

To Donn—With your help, the student has become a teacher.

To George and Iva—you have given me something to shoot for.

And thanks to you, the reader. I hope that this message makes a difference.

INTRODUCTION

You are about to learn concepts that may go against what you currently hold to be true. Many of the proven recommendations in this book fly in the face of mainstream dieting. This is because *The Fat-Fighter Diet* is not just about changing your eating habits. Rather, it is about taking control *of your life*. Success can be achieved only by approaching your body holistically. The very word "holistic" implies the importance of the whole and the interdependence of its parts. What you *think*, what you *eat*, and what you *do* each play starring roles in this movie called your life.

The Fat-Fighter Diet Will Improve Your Health and Well-being and What You See in the Mirror

Following *The Fat-Fighter Diet* will get you into the best physical shape of your life because this book begins with a focus on what you can't see—all of the tiny, daily thoughts and experiences that become years of imbedded learning about what you can and can't do; about how you feel about your body and the way you look; and about what you believe to be true about yourself and what you are capable of. The combination of a healthy mindset, proper nutrition, and physical exercise is the very essence of the holistic lifestyle you will learn about in the coming chapters.

The Fat-Fighter Diet Is about Health, Fitness, and Fat Loss, Not Simply "Weight Loss"

The Fat-Fighter Diet puts the focus where you need it—on *fat* loss. By following this program you will most likely lose weight; however, I can guarantee you will lose fat! These same principles are also essential for improving your health and increasing your level of physical fitness.

The Fat-Fighter Diet Is about Truth, Not Gimmicks

The truth is this: Lifelong health, fitness, and fat loss can be achieved only by balancing the three major contributors to your health:

1. Dedicate yourself to a mindset that reduces your stress and increases your focus on achieving and sustaining your goal.
2. Dedicate yourself to a delicious, alkaline-forming diet with the correct balance of protein, essential fats, and complex carbohydrates.
3. Dedicate yourself to prescriptive exercise. A triathlete will train very differently from a woman in her 40s looking to improve muscle tone and increase flexibility. Instead of a "one size fits all" exercise program, your plan should be designed according to your goal. Moreover, any weight loss or fat loss program that does not advocate exercise is dead wrong.

The Fat-Fighter Diet Is a Plan for Your Life—It Is Not a Quick Fix

The Fat-Fighter Diet has worked for thousands and it will work for you, but it will take some effort. Many of my clients own successful businesses that they built from zero. They didn't just wake up running a company; they built it from the ground up. This is the same way you will build your new body. Since it has taken you some time to get into the shape you are presently in, it will take some time to change. Owning your health and fitness is worth this small but powerful investment of time.

The Fat-Fighter Diet Designs a Program for You, Not the Same Program for Everyone

There are more than 6 billion people on the planet and no two are exactly the same. We all have different goals, body types, metabolisms, and are one of two genders, so why would we all follow the exact same fitness and nutrition program? With *The Fat-Fighter Diet* you will discover the exact food *you* should be eating, as well as the correct amount and types of exercises *you* should be doing for your body, your fitness level, and your goal.

The Fat-Fighter Diet Will Motivate You to Act and Not Just Read

Throughout this book you will find inspirational "action" statements that will prompt you to take action today. Now! *Actions*, not words, produce results.

The Fat-Fighter Diet Is Clear-Cut and Not about Guessing

Throughout each of the three sections of this book you will find tools to measure your progress. Measuring is the only way to know that what you are doing is producing the results you desire. Measuring your progress is quick, easy, and key to achieving your goals.

THE FAT-FIGHTER DIET HAS WORKED FOR OTHERS AND IT WILL WORK FOR YOU!

Earl Nightingale, the famous father of the self-help industry, once said that nothing great was ever accomplished without inspiration. To that end I give you three heroic examples that showcase exactly what can be achieved if you apply the principles outlined in *The Fat-Fighter Diet.*

SUSAN

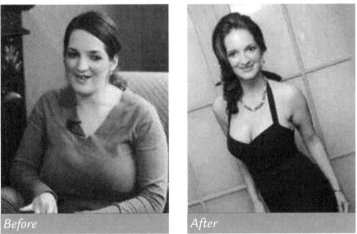

Before

After

Last fall I first met Susan, a waitress working at a local restaurant in the town of Oakville, Ontario where our personal training studio, BODiZONE, is located.

One of my clients, Dr. Stephen Thordarson, is a dentist with a practice in downtown Oakville. Dr. Steve, as I like to call him, is a skilled practitioner with a keen interest in cosmetic dentistry. Steve decided one day to hold a contest whereby one lucky Oakville resident would win a complete makeover from head to toe. Steve enlisted the help of our personal training company to take care of the fitness component while he and a few other practitioners would make over the winner's teeth, hair, etc.

Susan won that contest. She trained at BODiZONE for half an hour, three times per week using a combination of resistance training, cardiovascular training, stretching, and our on-line nutrition system. We also had Susan perform cardio sessions on her own two or three times per week for half-hour sessions. Out of 164 hours in a week, Susan spent only a total of three hours weekly using a combination of our nutrition, training, supplementation, and motivation to make the changes you see here.

Susan would be the first to tell you it wasn't the easiest thing she has ever done, but she will also tell you it is the *best* thing she has ever done. She set the goal and made it to the finish line. Bravo to you, Susan!

TONY

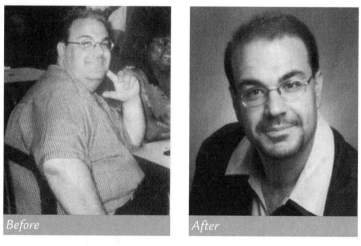

Before   After

Tony is a busy professional who works days, evenings, and weekends to reach his sales goals. Like many people, all the "diets" he had tried in the past had failed him. By cutting calories he would lose some weight, but quickly gain it all back a few short months later. Up until this point Tony had never seen the inside of a gym. As a matter of fact, he thought that weight training was only for "bulking up," something he was definitely not interested in doing!

We educated Tony on the importance of weight training as it relates to fat loss and introduced him to *The Fat-Fighter Diet* eating and supplementation approach. As a result, Tony slashed his body fat percentage and dropped several pant sizes. He has also developed the eating habits necessary to avoid diseases like diabetes and heart disease, which were gunning for him before.

Congrats to you Tony!

JACKIE

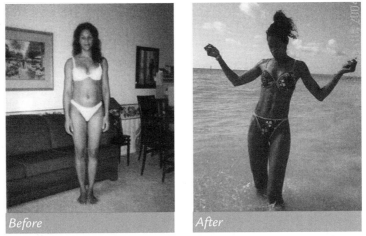

Before · After

Jackie is a busy mother who works full time and has a wicked sweet tooth! Her previous high carb- no-fat diet left her feeling sluggish, water retentive, and with very dry skin. After only four weeks using the Fat-Fighter nutrition and exercise program she had energy to spare and her skin was glowing. After twelve weeks Jackie had achieved all of her fitness goals. Way to go Jackie!

These are a small sample of the people who have made lasting changes in their lives using the Fat-Fighter Diet approach. For more examples, go to www.ebodi.com.

THE BOTTOM LINE

It is up to *you*.

No matter what your fitness level is today, you can change your body. By focusing on the areas of your life that you *can* control (what, when, and how much you eat; the frequency, duration, and type of exercise you do; how focused you are on achieving your goal; and the attitude and mindset you cultivate), you can achieve your ultimate fitness dream!

We have all read the statistics on weight management in North America. Over half of us are struggling with serious emotional and physical health issues directly related to our lifestyle choices. The power to change is yours alone.

If you are overweight and unhappy with yourself, it is up to *you* and you alone to make the changes necessary in order to achieve the body and health you desire. The moment you accept full responsibility for who you are is the moment you are ready to begin this program and start living the life you want in the body you deserve.

OUR BODY IS GUIDED BY OUR MIND

MINDSET
I will feed my mind only the best. I will become what I think about, all day long.

Each one of us is a marvel of creation; what Mother Nature has given you is truly beautiful. But stressful living, a poor diet, lack of supportive supplements, lack of sleep, inadequate activity, and environmental toxins build up over time, tarnishing that beauty. Although the Fat-Fighter Diet cannot change what Mother Nature has given you, it will provide you with a comprehensive plan to reverse the years of damaging habits, guiding you to become the best that *you* can be.

Everything you do and, ultimately, everything you become first begins with a thought. You are guided by your mind. In his now famous recording, "The Strangest Secret," Earl Nightingale said, "If you are ever going to change your life, you must change your thinking." The way you are thinking about yourself *right now* is forming the person you are becoming. Our lives and all of our experiences take place in our minds.

IT IS TIME TO THINK ABOUT WHAT YOU'RE THINKING ABOUT

The thoughts you choose to have each hour, each minute, and even each second throughout the day are directly affecting your behavior, self-talk, self-beliefs, decision making, goal setting, and focus. Together with your ability to manage stress, these factors will ultimately determine who and what you become both physically and emotionally. In *The Fat-Fighter Diet*, we will touch on each of these factors and discover why they are so important in changing your body and your health.

While the foods you eat and the exercises you do are vital to changing your physical body and improving your health, your mind is the master of all. We subconsciously move in the direction of our most dominant thoughts. In order to live a life full of energy and good health in a body free of disease and obesity, we must do what is necessary to obtain the results we desire. To accomplish this we must control our thinking, which in turn controls all of our actions. Before you can declare victory in "the battle of the bulge," you must *first* win the victory in your mind.

Self-Talk: We All Talk to Ourselves, But Are We Listening?

It is an unfortunate fact for most people that of the 80,000 plus thoughts they have in a day, 98 percent are the same as the thoughts they had yesterday, with most of these being negative. Have you ever really listened to what you are saying to yourself? Negative self-talk could be wreaking havoc on your mind and body. What you are thinking and the words you speak are subconsciously moving you in one of two directions—toward success or toward failure. Your words are self-fulfilling prophecies. If all you think about, talk about, and focus on is failure and negativity, why would you be surprised to see that you have failed? Conversely, if you focus on succeeding, it should come as no surprise when things "happen" to work out.

I am always amazed by the way people respond when asked how they feel about exercise. "I hate exercising" is one of the most commonly uttered statements along with "I hate broccoli!" The words you choose have the amazing ability to change "the color of your mind" and the way you feel *emotionally* about eating healthily and exercising. By making some subtle changes to the words you use when talking about exercise and nutrition, you will change the way you feel about your new lifestyle.

Instead of thinking "I will never lose this fat," try thinking "I am losing fat every day." Rather than saying to yourself, "I hate exercising," say, "Each time I exercise I am getting leaner and more healthy." Instead of thinking you can't do it, think of all the reasons why you can. These positive thoughts and words are to your mind what healthy food is to your body.

Think of your mind as a television with unlimited channels and a huge variety of programs to watch. If you find yourself focusing on something negative, simply use your mental remote control to change the channel. Please don't be like so many people who choose to pull up a chair, make some popcorn, and get comfortable with their negative thoughts. Focusing on negative mental programing can only bring about more negativity. Change the channel and focus on the positive.

Remember that your mind is a fertile ground of infinite possibility. Your potential is unlimited. You have the power within you to create the body and life you desire *starting today,* and it will not cost you a single cent.

Like a seed planted in good soil, your creative mind thrives in the field of positivism, and these thoughts give birth to the physical reality where we reside. It is a simple yet astonishing fact—your thoughts and words are creating your reality.

ACTION
Become aware of your thoughts and self-talk. When you find yourself thinking or speaking negatively, simply say to yourself "Next" and change your mental channel from something negative to something positive.

From Self-Talk Comes Self-Belief: Who Do You Think You Are?

> *For as he thinks within himself, so is he.*
> —King Solomon

In my business, I spend a great deal of time in a one-on-one setting with people. During this time I talk with my clients about all kinds of things—the weather, their work, their family, their friends, but mostly about themselves. Over the years I noticed something quite extraordinary. The people who spoke the most negatively were the same people who had the hardest time achieving their fitness goals. As a matter of fact, at the time of consultation I can pinpoint who is ready to achieve their fat loss and fitness goals and who will be held back from them! The reason for this boils down to something called *self-belief*. We define ourselves by who we *think* we are. Your self-belief is a culmination of your "I am" statements. This sense of certainty about who you are determines what you will (or will not) do.

- I am fat.
- I am unattractive.
- I am a failure.
- I am uncoordinated, and so on.

These "I am" beliefs are formed at various stages of our lives, starting in our childhood, and they ultimately form our identity. Everything you do and all you feel about yourself stems from your self-belief. This is the story you keep telling yourself, and if that story is negative, filled with doubt, or constructed of limiting beliefs, it is holding you back from having the body and life you desire.

When a person comes into my office and I hear negative "I am" statements, I know I have more to deal with than simply changing the client's eating and exercise habits. The first thing that *must* change is that person's *belief* about himself or herself!

One of the best methods to test your own self-beliefs is to get out a piece of paper and write the words "I am" followed by what feels true to you today:

· In terms of my fitness I believe I am:
· In terms of my health I believe I am:
· In terms of my relationships I believe I am:
· In terms of my finances I believe I am:
· In terms of my _____ I believe I am:

Take a long look at this list. Does it read negatively?

It is important never to define yourself as being something or someone whose qualities you do not want to possess. Always think of yourself as being that which you desire to become.

Thinking, speaking, and defining yourself as fat, out of shape, or lazy becomes a self-fulfilling prophecy and will quickly derail any chance of becoming the healthy, fit person you can be.

Now that you know this, I want you to make another list with the same "I am" statements followed by a blank space. Now, fill in this space with the "I am" statement of the person you *want* to be:

· I am attractive.
· I am in great shape.
· I am happy.
· I am successful.
· I am loved.
· I am sexy.

Isn't it amazing how much better it feels to write positively about yourself rather than negatively?

BEHAVE YOURSELF!

"You are what you do."

—Kuato

Your thoughts and beliefs are the catalyst to your habitual behaviors that ultimately form your life. Your behavior consists of all the things, big and small, that you do each day—when you get up, when you work out, what you eat, how you handle stress. All of your habitual behaviors have led you to the point where you are *right now*. Whether you need to lose body fat, gain lean muscle, or improve your overall health, your behaviors have brought you *here*. The good news is that by using the power of positive thinking and by implementing the following six steps, you can develop *new* behaviors that will take you wherever you want to go.

SIX STEPS TO PERMANENT CHANGE

You cannot get something for nothing.

—Napoleon Hill

Over the last decade of coaching people, I have identified six steps to permanently changing behavior:

1. *MAKE A DECISION:* Decide exactly who you *want* to be and write it down. Use positive words in the present tense, as though you are already this person. It is important that you believe in your heart and mind that you can become this new person you have decided to be.

   · I am _____
   · I own _____
   · I have _____
   · I earn _____

2. *VISUALIZE:* Visualization allows you to create a mental picture of what you want to happen as if it has already happened. To visualize is to think in pictures rather than with words. Because your brain thinks in pictures, it is important to vividly see yourself as having the body and living the life you want. In your mind's eye, see yourself as living and enjoying your newfound body and life. Become excited and emotional about it! Smile, laugh, cry, or do all of the above! The more emotions you can attach to your visualizations, the more real they become.

Visualization is a performance-enhancing technique used by coaches the world over. You may have heard of athletes visualizing their winning performance before the actual event. By doing so they are providing their subconscious mind with instructions that will cause them to automatically behave in a winning fashion.

A study by Soviet sport scientists discovered that 75 percent of visualization training combined with 25 percent of physical training had a greater impact on the performance of Olympic athletes than that of 25 percent of visualization and 75 percent of physical training. These findings are not limited to Russian athletes. The great American golf legend Jack Nicklaus writes, "I never hit a shot, not even in practice, without having a very sharp, in-focus picture of it in my head. It's like a color movie."

You do not have to be an athlete to enjoy the benefits of this training method. Start using this winning technique today and program your mind for becoming the person you want to become.

ACTION
Use your mind's eye to picture the person you want to be. Store this picture in your mind and recall it often.

3. *ACT:* You will often hear stories about Academy Award-winning actors actually "becoming" the character they are portraying in a particular film. Their winning performance is achieved only if they are able to be so convincing in their role that they actually trick themselves into thinking *they are* the person they are portraying. To be convincing, these actors will actually stay "in character" for weeks or months at a time!

Acting is something we all do anyway, so why not play a role you really love? Start acting the part of the person you want to become. Act the part of a fit person, a successful person, a happy person, or whatever person you wish to be. You may have heard the expression "Fake it until you make it." Great actors are known for "feeling" their way into a character. The reverse is also true—you can act your way into the person you wish to be.

ACTION

Begin acting the part of the person you want to be. Throw out the foods an "unhealthy" person would eat. Buy a gym membership just like a "healthy" person would do. Speak, think, and behave like this new person.

---

4. *BE CONSISTENT:* Practice makes perfect and it is only through repetition that we learn new skills. Doing something "once in a while" never produces dramatic results. This is no different. Act out your newfound role each day, preferably twice or more per day. Try to stay "in character" for as long as possible, gradually increasing the amount of time. Remember, your goal is to actually become and transform yourself into this new person you have decided to be.

ACTION

Stay "in character" more and more each day. The more often and longer you do this, the easier and more natural it will feel.

---

5. *USE PAIN AND PLEASURE TO YOUR ADVANTAGE:* It is important to realize that your mind will always move *toward* behaviors that are perceived to be pleasurable. Conversely, your mind will always move *away* from that which is perceived to be painful. This is the key to understanding why we engage in certain behaviors even when we know they are not good for us.

In order to consistently engage in positive behaviors, we need to *positively reinforce* the behaviors we know to be beneficial to us while simultaneously associating pain with those that are harmful. For many people, the reason they do not start a new lifestyle plan (like the one you are reading about now) is because they have tried other "diets" in the past only to meet with failure and disappointment (why these diets fail will be explained in detail in Chapter 5). Therefore, they are associating the pain of failure with a change in lifestyle and subsequently will never enjoy life in a healthy, fit body. Others may fear injury. These people will associate pain with exercise and avoid the gym like the plague!

Then there are the pleasure behaviors so many people are addicted to: smoking, drinking, drugs, sugar, and television. These folks associate these behaviors with pleasure and find it very difficult to cut down or quit. The key to changing behaviors is to associate pleasure with behaviors that move you toward your goal and pain with those that move you further away from your goal. How do you do that?

Perform this exercise. Write down five things you know you must do in order to improve your health and lose body fat. (This is the list of things you know deep down must happen for you to be lean and healthy.) Your list might read something like this:

1. I must start training with weights.
2. I must start doing regular cardiovascular exercise.
3. I must start eating three meals and two snacks daily.
4. I must start drinking eight to12 full glasses of water each day.
5. I must stop consuming white flour and white sugar.

Next, beside each of the above, write down the pain you associate with each of these actions. (This list should identify your fears.) Your answers might read like this:

1. Working out with weights hurts.
2. I do not have the time to do cardio on a regular basis.
3. I do not have the time to prepare all of those meals and I'm not hungry in the morning.
4. Drinking water is boring and makes me go to the bathroom too often.
5. All of my favorite foods contain white flour and sugar—everything else tastes bad.

Next, identify what will happen if you do not start doing those things you know you must do. (This list should scare you.) It might read as follows:

1. If I do not start training with weights, I will continue to lose muscle and further damage my metabolism and mobility.

2. If I do not start doing regular cardiovascular exercise, I will never burn the calories required to have the body and health I desire.
3. If I do not make the time to prepare and eat three meals and two snacks daily, I will never awaken my metabolism.
4. If I do not start drinking eight to12 full glasses of water each day, I will always retain water, have low energy, and feel mentally "foggy."
5. If I do not stop consuming foods that contain white flour and sugar, I will never burn off my fat and may develop type 2 diabetes. This in turn will lead to accelerated aging and decreased lifespan.

Lastly, write down the pleasure you will feel by implementing the necessary changes into your life. (This list should motivate you and get you excited!) Your list might read like this:

1. Training with weights will make me stronger, leaner, sexier, more youthful, more energetic, happier, and more optimistic. I will be able to beat my husband in an arm wrestle, outdo my son in a fitness test, and look 10 years younger.
2. Performing regular cardiovascular exercise will cause me to burn fat, strengthen my heart and lungs, lower cholesterol, make me look great in my jeans, increase the quantity (and quality) of my life, improve my mood and outlook on life, give me more energy and vitality, and add life to my years.
3. Eating three meals and two snacks daily will boost my metabolism and burn my body fat. This will also give me improved digestion, increased energy and decreased cravings, increase lean muscle tissue, and will enable me to eat foods I love all the time.
4. Drinking eight to12 full glasses of water each day will improve my skin tone and texture, increase fat burning, reduce water retention, increase strength, reduce appetite, and make me look and feel a whole lot better.
5. Cutting out white flour and white sugar will improve my cholesterol levels, dramatically reduce my chance of developing diabetes, strengthen my immune system, lose body fat, reduce the signs of aging, and give me a lot more energy! Plus there are other alternatives to sugar that taste just as sweet.

6. *DO NOT QUIT—EVER:* Quitting is not an option; you must persist and succeed. It is not realistic to think that if you plant a seed today, you will see a tree tomorrow! In his best-selling book *Think and Grow Rich*, Napoleon Hill says, "Before success comes to most people, they are sure to meet with much temporary defeat, and perhaps some failure. When faced with defeat the easiest and most logical thing to do is to *quit*. That is exactly what the majority of people do." This is what separates people who are successful from those who fail. In your quest to achieve your goal, you must never quit, no matter how many times you slip up. Babe Ruth, the famous baseball player, once held the record for the most home runs ever hit. The interesting thing is not how many home runs, but how many strikeouts Babe Ruth had. Over the course of his career, Babe hit 714 home runs. However, he also struck out 1,330 times—a near 2–1 ratio! Every successful life has chapters of failure. It is not "striking out" that matters; rather, it is what you do *after* that makes the difference.

ONLY *ACTION* PRODUCES RESULTS

There is immense power in changing your behaviors, altering your daily self-talk, and writing out positive affirmations that will do more than just make you feel better about yourself right now. You have created the groundwork necessary to *take action*. Action is required to produce change in every area of our lives, and action requires the power of our minds.

Now that your mind is positively supporting your efforts, ask yourself questions that will inspire you *right now* to take the actions necessary for becoming the healthy, fit person you want to be and for achieving your goals. But wait a minute, what *are* your goals?

GOAL SETTING: THE KEY TO BECOMING

2

Shoot for the moon. Even if you miss it you will land among the stars.
—Les Brown

It is in your moments of decision that your destiny is shaped.
—Anthony Robbins

The single biggest factor when determining whether a person will be successful lies in that person's ability to decide on exactly what it is that he or she wants. In other words, the biggest step to getting yourself into great shape or vibrant health is simply making up your mind and acting accordingly. When you make the decision that you will no longer accept your current body, life, or health, you have taken the crucial first step toward improving your life. The person you are today is the result of all the decisions you have made in your life up to this moment. Everything begins with a committed decision: It is not your destiny to always be overweight, to feel like your life is in limbo, or that you cannot get a break. If you are feeling this way, you simply have not made a committed decision to becoming who you really want to be. If you are not absolutely convinced that you need to make a change, then you might as well stop reading right now. Transforming your body and health will require total commitment and effort, and if you have not made the decision to stick with this program, you will probably fail. It is important to tell yourself that no matter what obstacles get in your way, you will remain totally committed to achieving your goal. Once you have this conviction, simply do the work required to get there. The world gets behind the woman or man with a plan. It is truly amazing. Once you decide what it is you want, the entire universe conspires to bring it to pass.

In a famous 1953 Harvard University study, researchers discovered that 3 percent of graduating students wrote down their fiscal goals for the future. Twenty years later, this class was revisited. The 3 percent who had written down their goals were worth more financially than the other 97 percent *combined*.

Goals are specific, measurable results that you would like to achieve *at a determined time in the future*. Goal setting is a proven and powerful success technique and it is crucial to directing your energy toward the tasks you wish to accomplish. Once you make the decision to set and achieve small goals, you will start to set *bigger* goals. Before you know it, you will be doing things you had never dreamed possible. Achieving goals creates an attitude of optimism, and the optimistic mind is a fertile ground for new opportunities. When you are positive and optimistic, you will attract more of the same into your life.

BRIDGING THE GAP

Whenever I go grocery shopping I pay attention to the foods that people are buying in the checkout line ahead of me. It comes as no surprise that the person who has a cart full of vegetables, fresh fruits, and lean proteins tends to be someone who is in good shape. Conversely, when a cart is filled with ice cream, frozen pizza, white flour products, and soft drinks, that shopper's physical body reflects those choices. The other day I observed such a person reading a well-known diet and fitness book, her cart filled with high-glycemic and refined foods. This person was also dressed in workout clothes, which led me to believe that she had an interest in improving her health and fitness. But why such poor food choices? Was I to accept the possibility that she had no idea that ice cream and soda pop are unhealthy food choices?

This woman, like millions of others, has not found a way of *bridging the gap* between knowing and doing. We all want to make positive changes, and we know to a certain degree what we should and should not be doing. Why is it that so many of us do not apply the knowledge we have learned? The answer lies in goals. Setting goals bridges the gap between knowing what to do and actually doing it.

Two Types of Goals

While all goals should conform to the SMART (specific, measurable, attainable, realistic, and timeframed) principle, there are two types of goals I want you to focus on to achieve success with the Fat-Fighter Diet:

1. Behavior goals
2. Outcome goals

Behavior goals are specific, focused activities that are required in order to achieve the larger outcome goal. You can't have one without the other.

Let's say your outcome goal is to lose 10 pounds of body fat. In order to accomplish this, you must become serious about your nutrition program. Perhaps you have fallen into the habit of eating before bed, which is keeping your fat loss on hold. In order to achieve your outcome goal (lose 10 pounds of fat), you must identify the behavior (eating before bed) that is keeping you from doing so. Once you have identified the problem, you can set a behavior goal of eating your last meal before eight o'clock in the evening, not right before bed.

Fat-Fighter Goal Setting

Take the time to identify and write down three outcome goals and six behavior goals:

·   My outcome goal #1 _____
·   My behavior goal 1a _____
·   My behavior goal 1b _____

·   My outcome goal #2 _____
·   My behavior goal 2a _____
·   My behavior goal 2b _____

·   My outcome goal #3 _____
·   My behavior goal 3a _____
·   My behavior goal 3b _____

NOTE: As you continue to read *The Fat-Fighter Diet* and become a fat loss expert, you will discover new information that may affect your behavior goals. Once you have finished reading this book, be sure to return to this section to review and update your behavior goals.

The Importance of Repetition

Now that you have identified your outcome and behavior goals, it is important that you read them twice per day to register them into your subconscious mind. Once registered, your subconscious mind, which is responsible for *autonomic* functions of your body such as breathing and heart rate, will then help guide you toward the achievement of your goals. When you read your goals, picture yourself as having already achieved them.

Read each goal with enthusiasm and passion. In addition, rewrite your goals once per week. The act of writing out your goals is an even more effective way of programing your subconscious than reading them.

Establish Accountability

Tell your friends, family, or coworkers about the goals you have just set. By telling people about your goals, you are establishing accountability for their achievement. Knowing that people close to you are aware of your intentions can be a powerful motivator when you are tempted to give up.

ACTION
Decide what you want to achieve. Identify and record your outcome and behavior goals. Read and rewrite your goals each day. Tell your friends about what you are going to accomplish. From this point on, your energy, your focus, and your life will be defined in relation to the goals you have just set.

YOU WANT IT, BUT WHY?

> *He who has a strong enough why can bear almost any how.*
> —Nietzsche

Now that you have set your goals, it is important to clearly identify *reasons* that support your goals. Most people would love to have a healthier, leaner, more energetic body, so why are they not doing anything about it? Do you think that these same people would take action if their doctor told them they will be dead in 90 days if they do not lose 20 pounds of fat? You bet! So why is that? Why does it always take something significant to move us to action? The answer lies in the reasons we use to justify our behavior.

When you attach powerful and motivating reasons for behaving a certain way, you get leverage and can follow through with that new behavior. For example, I know that if I do not get up tomorrow morning at 6:30 a.m., I will not be able to make it to my first training appointment at 8:00 a.m. If I am late or miss my appointment, I may lose my client, resulting in a loss of income (not good). This will also disappoint my business partner, who depends on me each day. Of course I would like to sleep in—that feels good at the moment—but the reason I have attached to getting up has given me the leverage I need to overcome my desire for extra sleep.

The key to achieving your goals lies in attaching *powerful, emotionally charged reasons* that support your new behavior. These reasons will then work to instill within you a burning desire to succeed. The more intense the desire, the greater the results.

QUESTIONS CREATE DESIRE

Do you value your health? Do you value your physical body? You've bought this book, so of course you do. Now, ask yourself why do you value your health? Why do you value your body? What would it feel like if you did not have the health you enjoy today? How would you feel if you had decreased mobility? Have you ever stopped to think about this?

Anyone who has ever visited or cared for people who are losing their health has experienced a heightened appreciation of their own well-being, mobility, health, and vitality. Acknowledging the reasons why you value your body and health will help create the leverage necessary to support you in the achievement of your goals. Ask yourself the following questions in order to help find *your* reasons:

· Am I happy with myself?
· Do I want a better life for myself?
· What will my health be like in one year if I do not make any changes?
· What will my body and health be like in five years if I do not make any changes?
· Do I love myself?
· Am I proud of who I am?
· Why do I want to change?
· How will I feel once I make the changes I desire?
· What will my life be like once I have achieved my goals?
· What will it feel like to have the body and health I have envisioned for myself?

Your answers to these questions contain powerful reasons for achieving your goals. Once you have identified these reasons, you will have given your goals strong support or "legs" on which to stand on. Next, I want you to write these reasons down in a notebook or wallet card together with your goals. Whenever you feel like binge eating, skipping workouts, or quitting all together, reread what you have written. The more you do this, the more often you will reinforce your positive, goal-achieving behavior, and the easier it will become for you. As a matter of fact, after a while it will become a part of your very being.

ACTION
Give your goals "legs" by identifying and writing down your reasons for achieving your goals.

DEADLINES = ACHIEVEMENT

At one time or another, especially through our childhood years, we all had *dreams*. Dreams filled our young imaginations with awe and excitement. Now that we are older, our dreams stay in the back of our minds and are not an actualized part of our lives. But why is this so often the case? Why is it that so many of us fail to have our dreams materialize? The answer lies in deadlines. You have heard it before: *Goals are dreams with a deadline.* It is one thing to say to yourself, "One day, I am going to have a lean and healthy body." After all, this is just a dream—there is no pressure to actually do anything about it. It is quite another thing to say, "In three months, I am going to have 15 percent body fat and a 28-inch waist."

Deadlines are perhaps the single most effective method of increasing productivity. Who hasn't put something off until the last possible minute only to complete the required task in a flurry of sudden productivity? This is the power of positive pressure through the use of deadlines. Once you attach a deadline to your dream of getting in shape, improving your health, or breaking a habit, you have transformed your dream into a goal.

ACTION
Set a definite deadline to achieving all of your behavior and outcome goals.

- I will achieve my outcome goal #1 by _____.
- I will achieve my behavior goal 1a by _____.
- I will achieve my behavior goal 1b by _____.
- I will achieve my outcome goal #2 by _____.
- I will achieve my behavior goal 2a by _____.
- I will achieve my behavior goal 2b by _____.
- I will achieve my outcome goal #3 by _____.
- I will achieve my behavior goal 3a by _____.
- I will achieve my behavior goal 3b by _____.

FOCUS POWER

The number one reason people fail is broken focus.

—Brian Tracy

Setting a goal is not unlike turning on the autopilot function of an airplane. Once you plant that goal in your mind, your subconscious mind will begin to steer you in the right direction. However, also like the autopilot function of an airplane, once you have set your course, you must continue to pay attention and monitor progress. It is important to remain alert and to guard against external forces that may distract you from your purpose. You must remain *focused* on achieving your goals.

Controlled focus is a powerful tool that can be used to break through any obstacle that is stopping you from achieving your goal. An example of the power of focus can be found by looking at the sun. On most days, each of us has the opportunity to go outside and bask in the light of the sun. Because the sun's rays are spread out all around us, we feel only the warmth upon our skin. However, if we take out a magnifying glass and hold it under the sun's light we can easily set fire to a piece of paper. When light is concentrated even more it becomes a laser beam with the ability to cut through steel. By focusing light, we are able to concentrate its power into a force to be reckoned with.

BECOME A FORCE TO BE RECKONED WITH

The most effective way I know to stay focused is to do something *every day* that will move you in the direction of achieving your goal.

Schedule time to go to the gym. Success is planned; failure isn't. Make a commitment to go to the gym by asking a friend to meet you or by hiring a personal trainer who will hold you accountable if you miss the appointment. Better still, record in your daytimer exactly when you should eat and exercise and hold yourself accountable for sticking to the behavior goals you have set.

Read motivational books and articles on health and fitness. Be sure to read something related to healthy, successful living each and every day. Choose materials that instruct and inspire you. It doesn't matter if this is a short article or an entire set of books—just read. By doing this you will continually refocus your mind on becoming and staying fit and healthy.

Go for a walk outdoors. Breathe deeply and swing your arms while you walk. Try to choose a path that takes you through a wooded area. Enjoy the sights and sounds of nature while you focus on your goals.

Purchase healthy foods from your grocery store. Go to your local organic garden center and purchase some fresh vegetables and fruits. In the summer, go to the organic fruit market and buy some delicious berries. In the fall, frequent a farmers' market for some fantastic fresh, seasonal produce. By purchasing healthy fruits and vegetables, you are focusing on the importance of feeding your body nutrient-dense, calorie-sparse foods.

Practise daily destressing techniques. Being stressed out does little to improve focus. Manage your stress with two proven stress-reduction techniques—prayer and/or meditation. Practise these time-tested stress reducers *daily* and feel the difference they will make in your life.

Spend time each day thinking about your goal. The garden of your subconscious mind will grow any thought you plant—it does not discriminate. Therefore, it is very important that you think only about what you want, not what you *do not* want. By focusing on what you want to happen, you are programing your mind to move in a positive direction.

ACTION
Focus *on doing something that will aid you in the achievement of your goal* every day. This will help to build momentum. Always think positively about your goal, as doing this will program your mind for success.

FAITH, THE FLIP SIDE OF FEAR

Faith is the grit in the soul that puts the dare into dreams.
—Robert Schuller

You have decided on your goals. You have written them down. You have given your goals "legs" to support them. You have set a deadline to achieving your goals. You are focusing on their achievement. Now what? Once you have planted the goal seeds in your mind, you must water them with *faith*. Faith is not religion. Faith is simply persistence. Faith is the flip side of fear, which would keep you frozen in one place forever. When you persist or keep working toward achieving your goal, you are demonstrating faith. If you did not have faith, you would never persist; you would give in to fear. In other words, faith is *expecting to succeed.*

As you go forward on this fat-loss journey, I want you to adopt the attitude that you can do it. You will succeed. Go out and buy an outfit that is two sizes smaller. Plan on attending your high school reunion. Buy a ticket for a beach vacation. Do these things with the belief that you will be fit and healthy when that day comes.

Whenever I talk about faith I am reminded of an individual who had so much faith that he changed the world of track and field forever. His name was Roger Bannister and the year was 1954. Roger had a dream. His dream was to run a mile in under four minutes at the summer Olympic Games. Up until that time, it was believed to be impossible, but Roger did not accept this. He believed that he could break the record. And break it he did. Roger did the impossible and ran the mile in three minutes, 59.4 seconds. Roger did not accept what everyone around him was saying. He expected to succeed and in doing so paved the way for others. Within 10 years of his accomplishment, no less than 336 other runners accomplished the same goal. But it took the faith of one person to break through the psychological barriers that were keeping others from achieving this goal.

So what are you to do if you do not have any faith? I have good news: Faith is abundant, free, and easy to acquire. All you have to do to possess faith is to *act as if* what you want is already yours.

- *Act as if* you are healthy by eating healthy foods.
- *Act as if* you are fit by exercising regularly.
- *Act as if* you are happy by remaining calm and cheerful and in the moment.
- *Act as if* you cannot fail by never giving up on achieving your goal.

William James, the great American psychologist, once wrote, "To feel brave, act as if we were brave." And this is what you must do.

Believe that you will succeed. *Act as if* you are already in possession of that which you seek. Stay in character each and every day and never quit. If you happen to falter in a moment of weakness, simply forgive yourself, refocus, and move on. This persistence—this *faith*—is what's truly necessary for your success.

The practice of deciding on, working toward, and achieving powerful, life-changing goals is a process that you can continue throughout your life. By doing so you are taking hold of the rudder that steers your destiny. It has been said that success is a journey and not a destination. I challenge you to focus on making your journey a trip to remember.

STRESS AND FAT LOSS: ACHIEVING PEACE OF MIND 3

You are too blessed to be stressed.

—Jewel Diamond Taylor

Managing our stress is a vital component to lasting health, long life, happiness, *and* fat loss. Recent studies have shown that approximately 40 percent of all North Americans suffer from stress-related adverse health effects. In addition, up to 90 percent of all doctor visits are for stress-related complaints or disorders. Stress has been linked to every leading cause of death, including cancer, heart disease, accidental death, cirrhosis, and suicide. Stress is also a major contributor to workplace absenteeism and decreased productivity. Studies have found that the most common health risk and major contributor of weight gain for obese people is stress. This is because obese people secrete more cortisol than people of an optimal weight, and cortisol activates fat-storage enzymes, which perpetuate their obesity.

However, stress is normal and each one of us experiences varying degrees of stress every day. Stress comes in many different forms. Some stressors, such as running late because of traffic, are relatively minor, while major, life-transforming events such as death, divorce, or the failure of a business can have a very significant effect upon our bodies and our minds. Trying to avoid stress completely is not realistic, nor is it advantageous. In fact, stress is an important part of everyday life. It is not possible to achieve positive adaptations and growth in any area of your life (physically or emotionally) without some form of stress to prompt them.

Exercise, for example, is a form of stress on the body. When done correctly and in the right amounts, it produces very beneficial outcomes. However, when done incorrectly or for prolonged periods of time, injury can result. What you want to avoid is *excessive* and *continuous* stress.

THE DHEA/CORTISOL BALANCE

Stressful events are a certainty for all of us, and the way that we interpret and internalize these events has a profound effect on two important hormones in our bodies, DHEA and cortisol. DHEA (or dehydroepiandrosterone) is a stress hormone produced by the adrenal glands. It is the most abundant of all of our hormones. DHEA is responsible for revitalizing, rebuilding, and restoring each of the over 100 trillion cells we have in our bodies. In nutritional researcher Sam Graci's book *The Food Connection*, he describes DHEA as the "mother hormone" because of its role in producing other adrenal hormones like estrogen, progesterone, and testosterone.

Cortisol is also a stress hormone produced by the adrenal glands. After DHEA, it is the second most abundant hormone. Cortisol is a glucocorticoid, meaning that it has the ability to increase blood glucose levels. This occurs as part of the fight or flight response, as cortisol assumes control of the body's metabolic systems during high-stress events. When faced with a life or death situation, cortisol will temporarily increase the flow of glucose (as well as protein and fat) out of your tissues and into the bloodstream. This increases physical readiness and energy in order to handle the stressful situation. However, when we prolong our stress through excessive worry, overwork, inadequate sleep, overtraining, and poor nutrition, cortisol's temporary job becomes a permanent one. When this happens, excess cortisol is produced, which raises insulin levels as well as blood pressure, reduces immune function, increases appetite and cravings for sugar, increases fat deposition (particularly around the abdominal area), and causes brain damage. Not a pretty picture. As you can see, it is very important that we keep cortisol in check.

Imagine that these two hormones, DHEA and cortisol, are seated on a teeter-totter with DHEA on one side and cortisol on the other. As one side goes up, the other side goes down. In order to keep our DHEA/cortisol teeter-totter from tipping too far to one side, we must remain in homeostasis, which is a state of equilibrium or balance. The more we can remain in balance, the healthier we will be both physically (by remaining disease free and in good physical shape) and mentally (by feeling happy and at peace).

When we spend our time worrying over our bodies, lives, jobs, etc., we are upsetting the DHEA/cortisol balance and damaging both our bodies and our minds. In many cases the solution is not to quit your job, go under the knife, or leave your relationship. This is like cutting off the head to cure the headache. Rather, the solution lies in finding practical ways to *manage* the stress that occurs each and every day.

EIGHT STEPS TO MITIGATE CORTISOL

Taking control of your cortisol levels can be achieved naturally using the following eight steps:

1. Avoid very low-calorie diets, especially for extended periods. The restriction of calories is a significant stress to the body, causing decreases in testosterone (in both men and women—yes, women have testosterone too, just less of it) and increases in cortisol.
2. Avoid overtraining (a common mistake). Keep workouts brief (less than 60 minutes) and intense by packing more work into less time.
3. Consume carbohydrates and proteins immediately following your workout. This will help to suppress the post-workout-induced stress response and maximize recovery.
4. Be sure to get seven to eight hours of deep, dark, restful sleep nightly (depriving yourself of sleep will raise cortisol).
5. Drink plenty of water (being dehydrated can raise cortisol).
6. Do not binge on alcohol.
7. Do not use stimulants such as caffeine or ephedrine.
8. Consume an alkalinizing diet (the more alkaline you are, the less cortisol you make—more on this in Chapter 8.

THE PEACE CONNECTION

Peace, the opposite of stress, is achieved through the realization that you are, first and foremost, a temporal being of peace. It is where you come from. You are not how you look or what you have. You are an energy force designed of love and from love. Peace in your life will be achieved by realizing this and reconnecting to this source. This reconnection to God or Nature or Love or Allah or Peace (whatever you would like to call it) is the only way to achieve permanent happiness and peace of mind. Everything else can and will be taken from you: Your body, your health, your friends, family, and possessions can all be stripped away.

But your connection to peace is always right there waiting for you to grasp hold of, anywhere, anytime. Sounds great, you say, but how do I connect with this force? I know of two fantastic ways: Prayer and meditation.

THINKING YOUR WAY THIN: MEDITATION AND PRAYER FOR STRESS RELIEF, HEALTH, AND FAT LOSS

Mindful prayer is not necessarily a religious activity, nor is it tied to any specific concept of God. Prayer is an outlet for expression, a communication with the world, the cosmos, that which is larger than you, and it allows you to identify feelings, thoughts, desires, dreams, disappointments, and successes. This "conversation with the Divine" is very cathartic and helps you to keep from bottling up your emotions and feelings.

Mindful prayer is also an excellent way of improving the mind-body connection and it helps to evoke a feeling of connectedness with other people and with the world. If you are interested in improving your IQ, then prayer may be just what you were looking for. Studies have proven that prayer will boost the brain neurotransmitter acetylcholine, resulting in improved intelligence. In addition to making you a "smarter" person, mindful prayer has also been shown to improve sleep, increase optimism, and elicit a feeling of having more than enough as opposed to not enough.

Meditation is another highly effective way to reduce stress and promote a healthy DHEA/cortisol balance. Using brain imaging, researchers have discovered that the simple act of meditation alters blood flow in the brain. When a person delves into a meditative state, blood flow is increased to the left prefrontal cortex. This is the part of the brain that is responsible for self-esteem, happiness, contentment, and peace.

According to Dr. Randy Knipping, B.Sc., MD, CCFP, and head of aviation and preventive medicine at the Cleveland Clinic Canada:

Meditation is the practice of developing understanding and acceptance of human nature through focused awareness of the mind and body. Meditation begins with drawing attention to the constant flow of thoughts, feelings, sensations, and experiences in a nondiscursive, nonanalytical, nonconceptual way. One simply watches, silently, observing passively everything that is, and simply accepting it as [it] is. There is no attempt to change, fix, transform, improve, develop, start, or stop anything.

Dr. Knipping explains:

Many who are new to meditation ask what the purpose is of meditation if one doesn't actually "do" anything at all. The simple answer is that we have been socialized from childhood to constantly "do something." From the moment we learn how to tie our shoes to the launch of a new business, it seems that we are being "successful" because we can measure success externally through well-tied shoes and profitable enterprises. But there is more to being human than being successful. What constitutes a good life is much about the relationships we have with ourselves and others. Loving kindness. Compassion. Equanimity. Peace. Meditation is about bringing balance back into your life. It is about breathing consciously, examining the flow of your life in real time, and not imposing upon the present moment that constant cacophony of action. Don't just do something, sit there (breathe, accept).

Dr. Knipping believes that mindfulness is a conduit to important lifestyle changes. "From this ocean of mindfulness naturally comes eating consciously, paying attention to food in such a way that overeating becomes impossible. There comes a natural observation that physical training results in an immediate sense of uplifting, energy, and stress resilience. There is less ego and more heart. There is life, and awareness of our precious human life. It is a beautiful practice."

Meditation is not hard work. You do not need to purchase any special equipment—not even candles are required! All you need is a quiet place where you can slow your mind and focus on your breathing. Like many things, at first meditating may seem a little awkward. After all, up to this point you may have thought this was something reserved for monks living high up in the mountains of Tibet! However, the importance of meditation is at an all-time high. With our fast-paced lives, high-stress demands, and inadequate nutrition placing huge stress on our bodies and minds, the practice of meditation has gone from something that we *should* do to something that we *must* do.

A PRIMARY MEDITATION TECHNIQUE

- Begin by sitting in a quiet place free from distractions. Adopt a comfortable but erect position. If you prefer, you can sit cross-legged on the floor or on a chair with your feet flat on the ground.
- The next step is to use the power of sustained focus of concentration to let go of any tension in your body.

- With a focus on the breath, concentrate on the cool sensation of inhaling through the nose and the warm, moist sensation of exhaling through the mouth.
- Allow your breathing to find its own rhythm. It may be useful to employ a word or phrase as a meditative focus. Silently repeat this word or phrase with each inhalation and exhalation.
- As you proceed, draw your attention to different areas of your body beginning with the lower extremities and moving upward. Search those areas for any tension and discomfort. With each inhalation gather any tension found into the breath and release the tension when you exhale.
- During your meditation your mind may wander. This is not uncommon and will improve with each time you meditate. If your mind does wander, simply bring your thoughts back to the breath.
- At the moment that you feel calm, peaceful, and tranquil, it is important to introduce a powerful intention. Ask that peace, love, health, equanimity, and gratitude flourish in your life. Inhale disappointments and exhale forgiveness.
- While in this meditative state, remain calm and listen. Feel gratitude and positivity flowing over and through you. Do not force this feeling—simply allow it to happen. Slowly inhale and exhale any control.

Ideally you should perform this meditation exercise for at least 20 minutes each day. In the beginning this may be unrealistic; however, even five minutes per day will make a difference. Meditation will becomes easier and more effective with practice, so emphasize consistency more than duration for maximum benefit.

ACTION

Manage your stress (and stress hormones) through daily meditation and the eight steps to DHEA/cortisol equilibrium.

DAILY SUCCESS HABITS

The following is a list of habits that, when practised daily, will produce staggering results. Some are actions while others encourage you to cultivate a state of mind. Read through each habit and while doing so think of ways to implement it into your life.

1. Gratitude

It is important for your mental health to take time each day to reflect on your blessings. Regardless of your present situation, you have much to be thankful for: your loved ones who support and care for you (no matter what your body fat percentage is); your family and friends whom you love; your senses, which allow you to see, hear, smell, taste, and touch; your body, which allows you to move, jump, run, or walk; your freedom to be whoever and whatever you decide to be. Thinking of all the things you have to be grateful for is an important reality check. Even the smallest bit of gratitude first thing in the morning (or any time of the day) will make a positive difference in your mind and your life.

The Gratitude Infinity Loop

Gratitude lends itself to being of service to others. Being of service to others in turn leads to fulfillment. This fulfillment leads right back to gratitude and the cycle repeats.

Begin your next day with a prayer of gratitude and see if it does not make a better day for you and for those around you.

GRATITUDE
Acknowledge every aspect of your
life that you are grateful for. Search
within yourself to discover all of
your miraculous blessings.

FULFILLMENT
Pay attention to the profound
sense of fulfillment that grows
from your Service—notice how
it nurtures your gratitude.

SERVICE
Apply yourself to those areas
that you believe in—devote
time and energy to things
beyond yourself.

2. Meditation

Reduce your stress and improve your DHEA/cortisol balance by putting into practice this age-old secret of peace. Meditation is easy and provides immediate results. Please see Chapter 3 for a meditation you can start using today.

3. Planning

You have heard it before: Failing to plan is planning to fail. This is true in many areas of life and particularly with your health and fitness. Regardless of whether your goal is to lose 10 pounds of body fat or to increase your mobility, you are going to have to plan exactly how to accomplish your goal. Write your plans down in a list and check off each accomplishment *each day*. This will give you tremendous satisfaction and immediate feedback as to how far you have come toward accomplishing your goals!

4. Exercise

Everyone agrees that we should all be exercising, and studies have shown a direct correlation between physical fitness and life fulfillment and success. Exercise can be fun and pays back huge dividends. In Chapter 17 you will be provided with all the information you need to begin your exercise program today.

5. Nutrition

You are what you eat. You have heard that before, but perhaps a more accurate statement is you are what you eat, digest, and assimilate. However you look at it, the fact remains the same: In order to have an energetic, high-performance body, you need to start feeding yourself high-performance fuel. A well-nourished and healthy body will out-perform an undernourished body just like a well-tuned engine will out-perform a poorly tuned engine. This performance enhancement will be both physical and mental, giving you a boost in all that you do, contributing to success in all of your endeavors. In Chapter 7 you will discover exactly what, when, and how much you should be eating in order to obtain a lean, healthy, and energetic body.

6. Valuing Time

Time is something we notice every day but rarely stop to really consider. We have all been assigned an unknown and finite amount of this precious commodity, yet many of us treat it with total disregard. Each day we all have the same amount given to us, and each day there are those who make the most of it and those who waste it. There are many thieves of time, but some of the worst offenders are watching television, surfing the Internet, reading tabloid magazines, snacking on junk food, bingeing on alcohol, and endless chatting on the phone. Lesser achievers often act as though they have 1,000 years to live by putting everything off until "tomorrow." Well, tomorrow rarely comes for these people. Do not become one of them. Start living the life you want *today*.

7. Sleep

This is a very important component to success in *every* area of your life. As a matter of fact, sleep is essential to life, just as water and food are. The old adage of needing seven or eight hours of sound, undisturbed sleep per night is very true. Your body does all of its repairing while you sleep. The muscles you stimulate during a workout do all of their growing and recuperating during deep, dark, restful sleep. Why dark sleep? This is beneficial due to the relationship between nature's light and dark cycles and our immune and metabolic energy systems. Our skin contains thousands of photoelectric cryptochrome cells. These cells interpret the amount of light photons we are exposed to, which in turn control the hormones prolactin, melatonin, and HGH (human growth hormone). These hormones are responsible for proper health and vitality. Melatonin is our most potent antioxidant source, which is our passport to remaining cancer free. Growth hormone, one of the body's master hormones, is responsible for strengthening bones, building muscle, decreasing body fat, and boosting the immune system. This means no clocks, nightlights, or flashing VCRs in your bedroom as they can all disrupt this important process.

Sleep is also important when it comes to fat loss. In a recent Nurses Health Study, researchers tracked more than 68,000 women for 16 years. These women were asked to report their weight and lifestyle regimen every two years. By the end of the study, the women who slept five hours each night were 32 percent more likely to experience major weight gain—defined as an increase of 33 pounds or more—and 15 percent more likely to become obese, compared with women who slept seven hours. And women who slept for six hours were 12 percent more likely to experience major weight gain and 6 percent more likely to become obese over the study period compared with women who slept seven hours a night.

In order to have optimum recovery of all of your bodily systems, you should adhere to the following sleep guidelines:

· Go to sleep early in the dark cycle each night and avoid staying up too late.
· Do not eat high insulin-producing foods (refined white flour, sugar), especially in the evening. These insulin-raising foods will shut down melatonin secretion. Melatonin is a powerful anti-cancer hormone.
· Do not consume excess calories.
· Go to bed at the same time every night.
· Reduce stress and do not watch television in bed as studies have shown this to increase stress. Reserve the bedroom for sleep and intimacy.
· Avoid caffeinated beverages after the early morning.
· Ensure that daily vitamin and mineral intake is adequate.
· Go to sleep in complete darkness. Block out all light from extraneous sources like street lamps, clock radios, alarm clocks, etc. Light can also interfere with melatonin secretion.
· Get seven or eight hours of sleep each night.

8. Learning

Continual learning is a tremendous success habit. Og Mandino, author of *The Greatest Salesman in the World*, once said, "You will be the same person in ten years as you are today except for the people you meet and the books you read." We should all strive to continue learning and to expand our minds. It is incredible to see the changes that can occur in people's lives when they broaden their horizons by becoming more educated. Have an open mind to learning new concepts and new ways of doing things. In the 1980s the belief was that all fat was bad. We now know that to be completely false. Essential fatty acids are very important and are included in a healthy, well-rounded diet. Twenty years ago that would have seemed crazy, but today it is accepted as a truth. By continuing to learn and ask questions, you will expand both your abilities and your possibilities.

9. Having Fun

One thing is for sure—we all need to have fun in our lives. Do not make this new lifestyle drudgery. Instead, find enjoyment in your healthy meals, knowing that you are fueling your body's fat loss, muscle growth, recovery, and healing processes. Take pleasure in your workouts, knowing that there are thousands of people who would give anything to have the mobility and freedom of movement that you enjoy. Find a friend to do your program with and enjoy some friendly competition while supporting and encouraging each other to victory. Smile and find the pleasure that is in the process of being successful.

10. Control Emotions

Be a master of your emotions—do not let them be the masters of you. This is very important if you wish to remain calm and on track. Do not let little things upset you and get you off course. Sometimes people use a small "crisis" as a reason to skip workouts and eat junk food. This will only cause the problem to be magnified. Instead, try another approach: Smile when you are angry, work when you are tired, and laugh when you feel stressed. By taking control of your emotions, you empower yourself to achieve your goals without wasting precious energy unnecessarily. You also create calmer waters within your life, which is more likely to attract the same from others. Try it!

11. Honor

"Honor" is a very serious word. To honor someone means to respect others' wishes and well-being. We are told to honor our mother and father and each other. However, we must also honor ourselves. To honor yourself means to not take your health, body, mind, spirit, and mobility for granted. Treat yourself with respect and honor by not polluting your body or mind with garbage foods and negativity. Follow your meal plans, exercise consistently, practise the daily success habits, and surround yourself with positive people and positive thoughts. Do this and you will see the world change before your very eyes. Your life will become an example for others to follow.

12. Support

This may just be the most important success habit of all.

Find and cultivate a supportive social network of friends, colleagues, and mentors with whom you can share your health and fat loss thoughts, challenges, and experiences.

For many people, the challenge of starting and sticking to a change in dietary and lifestyle habits can initially be overwhelming. Long-term studies examining the relapse rate of people who lost weight found that 90 percent do not keep it off because they do not have the necessary long-term support and accountability. According to a study by the American Association of Naturopathic Physicians (AANP), 90 percent of people who attended at least half of their weight-loss support meetings kept their weight off. In comparison, of those participants who were self-monitored with no support system, a staggering 100 percent regained their weight! This study and others give credence to the fact that while it is up to you to do the proper exercises and eat the right foods, you should not do it alone. Reach out to those who share your desire for improved health and fitness. Tell them about this book and what you are going to achieve. Together you can share the motivation and experience of learning to take control over your health, body, and life.

13. Commitment

Are you ready to commit to achieving your goal body fat percentage, to maximizing your health, and to owning a truly fit body? Are you ready to do *whatever it takes* each and every day until you succeed? A true commitment means there is no turning back. There is no way out. It is to adopt the mindset that you are going to do this no matter what! If you are not feeling this sense of conviction, I suggest that you go back and reread this section again. With the power of commitment there are no obstacles too big, no challenges so foreboding that you cannot overcome! I am ready if you are!

ACTION
Make the preceding success habits a part of your everyday routine.

TRANSFORM WORDS INTO ACTION!

To-Do List:

- Determine what you want to accomplish.
- Set your behavior and outcome goals.
- Set deadlines for their achievement.
- Practise daily stress-management techniques.
- Follow the daily success habits.
- Persist until you succeed.

After reading this first section, I hope you have come to accept the importance of your mind as it relates to fat loss and achieving your fitness goals. You have learned how what you think about each moment of each day is constantly determining your behavior, self-talk, self-beliefs, goal setting, and focus, and how these factors are forming the person you are today as well as the person you will become tomorrow. You have also discovered why it is important to manage your stress if you wish to be both lean and at peace. Most importantly, you know that becoming fit and healthy is a decision that only you can make. We must all take the time to decide on exactly who and what we want to become. The decision to live your life in a healthy, fit body with a clearly defined purpose is yours and yours alone. It is in these moments of decision that our lives are formed.

In the next section, I will show you how the decisions you make regarding what, when, and how much you eat are forming the person you are today and the person you will become in the future. I will illustrate for you why low-calorie diets are not the answer, as well as the right way to measure your progress.

In Phase One of the diet plan, you will discover the importance of cleansing as it relates to your overall health and body fat reduction. In Phase Two, I will explain exactly what, when, and how much you should eat in order to achieve your goal. You will learn why some foods are worse than others and the truth about carbohydrates, proteins, and fats. I will also provide you with goal-specific supplement recommendations that will help you achieve better results faster.

Later in this book, I will explain why exercise is so important when embarking on a weight loss journey and provide you with a detailed, personalized exercise plan to get you results fast and keep the results for life.

Regardless of your age or physical condition, it is never too late to start living a holistic, healthy lifestyle. The body is highly adaptable. Given the right combination of a healthy mindset, prescriptive nutrition, and proper exercise, your body can and will regenerate and thrive. By implementing the mental techniques and philosophies discussed in this section, as well as the nutrition and fitness strategies discussed in the next, you are well on your way to living your new holistic life.

THE FAT-FIGHTER *UN*-DIET: WHY MOST DIETS FAIL

MINDSET

Food is my friend. With every healthy meal I have an opportunity to make myself fit, healthy, and satisfied.

Your "diet" is quite simply the foods and beverages you consume, nothing more and nothing less. The word "diet" does not necessarily mean something good or something bad. In fact, the word "diet" is rooted in Latin and means "a way of life." I have met people who are on the McDonald's Diet, the "whatever I want" diet, as well as the Atkins, Bernstein, and South Beach diets, to name but a few.

As I mentioned earlier, the Fat-Fighter Diet is not intended to be something that you follow for a short period of time and then forget about. Rather, it is a plan to optimize your health, fitness, and life. By motivating and educating yourself to make better choices when you eat, you are creating a new lifestyle that will move you beyond simply calorie counting and into a whole new way of living.

Conventional dieting, as prescribed in all mainstream diet books, will have you believe that if you simply eat less you will lose weight. Need to lose a bit more? No problem! Cut the calories again. But when does this end?

Author Rob Faigin, writing in the book *Natural Hormone Enhancement*, makes this interesting observation: "If there existed an airtight mathematical relationship between caloric intake and weight loss, cutting caloric intake from 3,000 to 1,000 would result in a 730,000 calorie per year deficit—and would result in a 200 pound weight loss after a year. What if the person began the diet weighing 200 pounds? Would he disappear?"

Most of the popular diets today advocate a very low level of calorie consumption. These low-calorie diets usually elicit an initial weight loss of a few scale pounds, most of this being water weight. This initial weight loss is, of course, encouraging to the unsuspecting dieter. They naturally assume that this is fat loss, and that they are off to a good start. But what is really happening here? What do low-calorie diets really do to your body?

EFFECTS OF LOW-CALORIE DIETS

1. Low-calorie diets cause you to lose muscle. This is the worst thing that can happen to a person looking to lose body fat. When you consume too few calories, your body kicks into survival mode. Sensing that a famine is near, your body promptly disposes of its most metabolically active (and calorie-consuming) tissue—muscle. It does this through a process called gluconeogenesis, which is essentially the conversion of muscle to glucose for energy. You may be wondering why this is bad. After all, you are still losing weight. The problem is that when you lose muscle mass, you are subsequently decreasing your metabolic rate. The minute you even slightly increase your calories again, you immediately start packing on the pounds. This slowing of the metabolism is the reason why people tend to lose and gain weight in a yo-yo fashion with conventional dieting.

2. Low-calorie diets make you feel sluggish and tired. This is problematic for two reasons:
   · When you are feeling constantly tired and run down, you are very unlikely to be able to keep up with your resistance training and cardiovascular exercise routines, both of which are vital for long-term health and fat loss.
   · Low-calorie dieting has a negative psychological effect. Because you are denying yourself calories that your body actually needs, you are developing a negative relationship with food. Food is not the enemy: It is an essential source of natural healing, energy, and life.

3. Low-calorie diets cause your body to increase fat-storing capabilities, as fat is the best form of sustained energy in what your body perceives to be a time of famine. When you reduce your calories too low, your body starts to make more of the fat-storing enzyme lipoprotein lipase or LPL. This causes your body to convert more of the calories you consume into fat.

4. Low-calorie diets will decrease thyroid (T3) output. Your thyroid gland aids in regulating your metabolism, the series of chemical reactions taking place in your body that are responsible for creating energy and burning calories. When your calories drop too low, your body will reduce the output of T3, slowing your metabolism for further energy conservation.

FAT LOSS VERSUS WEIGHT LOSS

Question: Which weighs more—a pound of muscle or a pound of fat?
Answer: They both weigh the same, of course. A pound is a pound.

Question: Which is bigger—a pound of muscle or a pound of fat?
Answer: The pound of fat is bigger. Fat is less dense than muscle and therefore takes up more space on our bodies.

Question: Is there a difference between fat loss and weight loss?
Answer: There is a huge difference. Losing weight is actually quite easy. I have seen people lose more than 5 pounds of water in a single day. But losing body fat is an entirely different story.

LOSE 20 POUNDS IN 20 DAYS!

We have all seen the ads; some of you may even have tried out the "program." Some of you probably lost weight as well. But what did you really lose? Let's look at a typical scenario:

Subject A (before diet)
- 150 pounds
- 30 percent body fat
- = 45 pounds of fat, 105 pounds of lean body mass

This person decides to go on a low-calorie diet. After three months she has lost 20 pounds. These are her new stats:

Subject A (after diet)
- 130 pounds
- 28 percent body fat
- = 36.4 pounds of fat, 93.6 pounds of lean body mass

At first glance you may think that this person has succeeded. After all, she is 20 pounds lighter, but look closely. We can see that while the scale weight has gone down, her body fat percentage has not changed much. Worst of all, her lean body mass has actually gone *down*. Why is this important? Let's flash forward three more months. It is usually after this period of time that most people have abandoned their low-calorie diet and have relapsed back into their old eating habits.

Subject A (three months later)
· 150 pounds
· 35 percent body fat
· = 52.5 pounds of fat, 97.5 pounds of lean body mass

As you can see, she has not only returned to her original weight, she has actually gained body fat and lost muscle—exactly the opposite of what you want to do. This loss of muscle mass has further slowed her metabolism, making it harder for her to lose fat in the future—and a whole lot easier to gain more of it back. This is why conventional diets do not work. Any diet that sacrifices muscle tissue in the pursuit of weight loss is fundamentally flawed and doomed to failure.

ACTION
To ensure success, focus on health, fitness, and fat loss, not simply weight loss.

KEEP YOUR MUSCLES
The consequences of sacrificing muscle mass in the pursuit of weight loss are extremely serious and include:

· Back pain
· Cancer
· Diabetes
· Estrogen imbalance
· Excess fatigue
· Heart disease
· High cholesterol
· Metabolic syndrome
· Osteoarthritis
· Respiratory problems
· Sleep apnea
· Stroke
· Urinary incontinence

This is why it is so important to monitor your progress while following an exercise and nutrition program. It is only through monitoring that you will truly know whether you are changing your body composition in the right direction by burning fat and building muscle.

Monitoring Progress

When you are trying to change your body composition, it is important that you track your progress the *right* way. While most diets will have you monitor your body weight, as I mentioned earlier, body weight alone is a poor indicator of your overall state of health and fitness. Keep in mind that while more than 65 percent of the U.S. adult population are overweight and 30 percent are obese, approximately 20 percent of these people may not realize that they need to lose excess body fat because they appear to be of normal weight. However, despite looking "normal," these people have unhealthy body composition with an unacceptable muscle-to-fat ratio. It is only through the monitoring, measuring, and recording of your *body fat percentage* that you will truly know whether or not a fat-loss program is working for you. There are several ways of doing this, but the following three are by far the most accurate and most accessible:

1. You can use a mathematical equation based upon body measurements, height, and weight. (You can find a free tool that does this on www.ebodi. com. Simply click on the Free Wellness Analysis and your results will be sent to your inbox.) This method is quite accurate and is used by the U.S. Navy. I recommend dating and recording your measurements in a diary or logbook so that you can watch the numbers decrease over time, which is ultimately what matters most.

2. You can use skin-fold calipers. When done correctly, this is the preferred method of choice. Most body fat is stored subcutaneous or beneath the skin. By using skin-fold calipers to pinch folds of skin and fat at precise areas of the body, a skilled tester can determine with great accuracy the body fat percentage of a man or woman. Because of the personal nature of skin-fold testing, try to find someone skilled whom you trust to accurately measure your progress. This is time well spent since using an accurate testing method will allow for you to track even slight changes in your body composition.

3. Infrared (Futrex). This device sends a beam of infrared light into your biceps muscle. Fluctuations in the wavelength of the beam are used to estimate body fat percentage. One of the great things about this method is the ease of use—it is a breeze! The popularity of this method is increasing and many health professionals now have them in their office. Ask your doctor, chiropractor, or other health care professional to test you.

A Note on the Body Mass Index

The body mass index (BMI) can be defined as a measure of body fat based on height and weight that applies to both adult men and women. The problem with BMI is that it does not take into account fat versus lean tissue. The BMI incorrectly diagnoses about 25 percent of the population and is completely useless for athletes. For example, I know an athlete who is 6 feet tall and weighs 205 pounds. According to his BMI of 27.8, he is overweight. However, he has only 8 percent body fat and is in great shape. Forget about the BMI and focus on body fat percentage instead.

ACTION
Get your body fat tested and record your results. Monitor your progress by retesting every four to six weeks.

WHAT PERCENTAGE DO YOU WANT TO BE?

You are probably asking yourself what percentage you should be. Take a look below to see how you measure up.

	Men	Women
Extremely lean (body builder)	3–6%	9–12%
Very lean (fitness model)	< 9%	< 15%
Lean (beach body)	10–14%	16–20%
Average (good shape)	15–10%	21–25%
Below average	21–25%	26–30%
Needs improvement	26–30% +	31–40%

Before we begin talking about what, when, and how much you should eat, I want to make sure that you have clearly identified the body fat percentage you would like to be. The amount of time it will take you to reach this goal will depend on how much you have to lose. A realistic goal is to shoot for losing about 2 percent per month. At this rate you are unlikely to be losing muscle mass. Therefore, if you are currently 30 percent body fat, you will need about five months to reach 20 percent.

I would like to encourage you to keep accurate records of your progress. In addition to monitoring your body fat percentage, I would also suggest that you do the following:

- Take a "before" picture of yourself. Take another picture (using similar lighting and clothing) every 30 days. Pictures will often show progress that you just do not notice by looking in the mirror every day.
- Take measurements. Measurements are an excellent indicator of progress. Measure and record the following every four to six weeks:

Men	Women
Waist	Waist
Chest	Hips
Shoulders	Shoulders
Upper arms (biceps)	Upper arms (biceps)
Thighs	Thighs

Special Note Regarding Waist Circumference

Recent research has discovered that your waist circumference is an excellent predictor of morbidity. If at the age of 50 you have a waist circumference of 44 inches (female) or 45 inches (male) you have roughly the same chance of premature death as if you had breast or prostate cancer!

ACTION

Take the time to record and track your progress. This type of monitoring will tell the true story about your progress, while relying solely on the scale will only leave you feeling disappointed in the long run.

Knowing how to track your progress is a vital component to success in any endeavor. Having the ability to reflect upon how far you have progressed will fill you with a renewed sense of conviction that you not only *can* do it, you actually *are* doing it! Please keep this in mind as we move on to the next chapter and discover how you should prepare to propel yourself toward your goal!

PHASE ONE: PREPARE

While you are embarking on your new Fat-Fighter Diet lifestyle, it is important to remember that you are now eating for the body you want, *not* the body you have. The way you have been eating in the past has largely contributed to the shape that your body is in today. If you continue to eat this way, you will not see a dramatic and lasting change, even if you begin to exercise. Your food choices and meal frequency will contribute approximately 80 percent *or more* to the way you look and feel.

Your body is in a constant state of renewal. In one year, the over 100 trillion cells that make up your bones, hair, teeth, organs, muscles, blood, and brain will all be new. Your body regenerates itself with the help of the building materials you supply it with. You are the general contractor! It is up to you to make sure that this new body of yours is built using only the finest materials. If you were building your dream house, would you allow the contractor to use substandard materials that were not up to code? Absolutely not. So why would you treat your body any differently? After all, you can burn your house to the ground and completely rebuild it. But once your body breaks down and wears out, that's it. You don't get another one.

Your current food habits have brought you to where you are today. However, as you now know, in as little as 21 days your body can form new habits. For this reason, be sure to give the first three weeks of this program your very best effort.

There are two phases in the Fat-Fighter Diet. In Phase One, you will *prepare* your body and your kitchen through cleansing. In Phase Two you will *propel* yourself toward your goal by discovering exactly how much, how often, when, and what you should be eating.

PREPARE: CLEANSING YOU KITCHEN

Take a walk through your kitchen. Open all of your cupboards as well as your fridge and take a good look at exactly what foods are lurking inside. Are there sugary snacks, boxed cereals, baked goods, cookies, sweets, junk foods, and other nutrient-sparse, calorie-dense foods waiting to tempt you in a moment of weakness? If so, throw them out! As Dr. Phil likes to say, "You can't eat unhealthy food if it's not there." The easiest way to avoid succumbing to a craving is to make it as difficult as possible to cheat. We all have lapses in willpower. The media does not help by bombarding us with commercials of high-fat, high-sugar meals day after day. Do not give yourself a choice. In the beginning of this journey your willpower will be at its weakest. Make it easier on yourself by throwing out these high-temptation food items. Each time you do not succumb to your craving, you will give your willpower muscles a workout, strengthening them for future battles.

ACTION

Eliminate access to those foods that you know are unhealthy and day by day you will feel your cravings gradually disappear. Then replace these items with healthy, nutrient-dense, low-calorie options.

PREPARE: CLEANSING YOUR BODY

Once your kitchen is ready, you will embark on a seven-day cleanse. During this period you will switch your metabolism from sugar-burning to fat-burning. During this phase you will eliminate certain foods while introducing others.

Why Cleanse?

In today's modern world, we are exposed to toxic substances all around us. We are bombarded with pollutants in the air we breathe, and with pesticides and fungicides on the food we eat and in the water we drink. We ingest toxic residues from medications and processed foods, and toxins build up from daily stress.

The human body is highly adaptable; however, the constant effect of so many toxic substances over long periods can wreak havoc on the liver, intestines, kidneys, lungs, and skin, which are the organs that facilitate the detoxification process. If these organs get backed up with too many toxins, it impedes them from doing their regular jobs, and contributes to disease processes. Toxic buildup can cause both psychological and neurological symptoms such as depression, mental confusion/fog, fatigue, headaches, irritability, tingling in the hands and feet, poor coordination, impaired nervous function, lowered immunity, allergies, and increased rates for many cancers. It can also contribute to skin breakouts and weight gain. Lending support to our detoxification organs will greatly improve overall health and also help boost the fat-loss process.

The liver is one of the main organs for detoxifying pollutants and chemicals in the body. It is also responsible for fat metabolism. Supporting the liver will help improve fat metabolism and increase fat loss. Research published in the *International Journal of Obesity* indicates that liver toxicity can often lead to excess body fat accumulation. Moderately obese people frequently suffer from liver dysfunction.

Many toxins are stored in the large intestine. It is believed that toxins in the intestinal tract irritate the intestinal membrane, causing it to produce a mucus coating as a form of protection. Over time this mucus coating thickens, preventing the toxins from being absorbed. The problem is that this coating also decreases the absorption of nutrients.

By engaging in a healthy detoxification process, you will help the body eliminate stored toxins, improve digestion, ensure a healthier metabolism, lose weight, and improve overall health.

I recommend an easy-to-follow one-week cleanse. This is not to be confused with fasting or a liquid diet, which was used in the past to give the digestive system a break. Fasting can be dangerous for people who suffer from hypoglycemia or diabetes as it can greatly disrupt blood sugar levels. Also, fasting can be counterproductive for fat loss for the same reason that low-calorie diets are doomed to fail. When you eliminate food, the body goes into "starvation adaptation" mode. Our bodies are hardwired for survival, and when there is an absence of food, we go into fat-storage mode. This was a highly beneficial adaptation response in the era of hunters and gatherers as it promulgated survival during times of famine. When food is introduced again, it will be promptly stored as fat because the body is anticipating famine.

The Seven-Day Quick Cleanse

This is an easy-to-follow plan that will support the digestive system (without triggering a fat-storage effect) as well as the detoxification of organs. This will get you on track to achieving improved health, energy, and fat loss. This is a great start to any fat-loss plan. In fact, most people will start losing fat right away.

Foods to Eliminate

1. Eliminate All Processed and Refined Foods

Most processed and refined foods lack nutrient value and yet are high in calories and trans fats. They are filled with additives, taste enhancers, sugar, artificial sweeteners, preservatives, and loads of chemicals that we can hardly pronounce, let alone digest. All these additives disrupt your hormonal balance, and leave your cells deprived of nutrients. Even some foods traditionally thought to be healthy, such as rice, pasta, and bread, are often overprocessed. These foods have often been refined or stripped of their fiber and nutrient content, bleached, and packaged for a long shelf life. Overconsumption can lead to many health concerns such as weight gain, digestive problems, fatigue, hypoglycemia, skin disorders, and many other common ailments. In general, look for 100 percent whole-grain bread and pasta products, which are higher in fiber and nutrients, and will help to keep your blood sugar levels balanced. Using brown or black rice, as opposed to white, is another great way to enjoy the foods you love without experiencing the detrimental effects of overprocessing.

Processed foods are attractive to many people because they are convenient, but is it worth trading convenience for health? It is a good idea to limit or omit processed and refined foods from your diet completely, but for the purpose of this cleanse, you will need to completely eliminate them for seven days.

Foods to Eliminate
· all white baked goods—muffins, cakes, cookies, white bread, doughnuts
· processed cereals, granola bars
· refined grains—white rice, white pasta, quick-cook oats
· all foods containing food additives: artificial colors, flavors, preservatives, sweeteners, texturing agents
· frozen dinners, prepackaged meals
· all foods containing sugar or artificial sweeteners

Foods to Enjoy
· whole rolled oats
· brown rice
· brown rice pasta
· 100 percent whole-grain bread

- black rice
- wild rice
- 100 percent whole-grain pasta

2. *Eliminate Dairy*

Many people consume dairy products for their high calcium content. However, studies have shown that North Americans are the highest consumers of dairy, but they also suffer from the highest incidence of osteoporosis. The reason for this is that dairy is an acid-forming food, and when the body is too acidic, it will leach calcium from the bones to act as a buffer. Better sources of calcium during (and after) the cleanse include sesame seeds, almonds, sunflower seeds, soybeans or soy milk, broccoli, spinach, salmon, and slow-cook oatmeal. You will learn more about blood acidity and fat loss in Chapter 8, "The Acid-Alkaline Connection."

Dairy contains many of the most common food allergens, and may also contain trace levels of antibiotics and hormones, which can disrupt the digestive and hormonal system.

Lactose intolerance is also an issue for a large portion of the population. In fact, between 30 million and 50 million Americans are lactose intolerant, with certain populations being more affected than others. Up to 80 percent of African Americans, 80–100 percent of American Indians, and 90–100 percent of Asian Americans are lactose intolerant.

It is also interesting to note that no other animal on this earth drinks milk as a normal part of their diet after being weaned, let alone the milk of another animal. The protein content in cow's milk is often difficult for us to digest and, as a result, contributes to increased inflammation and mucus, particularly in the digestive tract. This disturbance can lead to various health problems, including the following:

- allergies
- asthma
- acne
- dark circles under the eyes
- digestive complaints such as bloating and diarrhea
- ear infections
- weight gain

Foods to Eliminate
- · all cheese
- · all milk
- · yogurt
- · cream
- · ice cream and frozen yogurt
- · any dips or sauces with dairy as an ingredient

Foods to Enjoy
- · soy, rice, or almond milk
- · soy or rice cheese
- · soy yogurt

Organic dairy, such as yogurt or rice, can be introduced in Phase Two.

3. *Eliminate Red Meat*

There are many health reasons to avoid eating red meat. The saturated animal fat in red meat contributes to heart disease and arteriosclerosis. It can cause inflammation in the intestinal tract, contributing to bowel disease. A new study published in the *Journal of the American Medical Association* (JAMA) shows a doubling of the risk of colon cancer for people who are heavy consumers of red meat. Red meat is acid forming, and overconsumption will disrupt the desired alkaline state that is necessary for a healthy and lean body.

In addition, red meat can contain contaminants such as heavy metals, pesticides, and undesirable environmental pollutants that tend to collect in the fat tissues of animals, which are then absorbed into your body. If you absolutely must eat red meat, do so sparingly and only in Phase Two of the diet.

Foods to Eliminate
- · beef
- · lamb
- · pork
- · rabbit
- · veal
- · venison

Foods to Enjoy
- · beans and legumes
- · cold-water fish
- · free-range chicken and turkey
- · free-range eggs
- · raw nuts and seeds
- · tempeh
- · tofu
- · whey or soy protein isolates

While the elimination of certain foods is necessary during the cleanse, it should be noted that the following foods must be consumed for maximum benefit. Increasing your intake of these foods will ensure that all toxins being released during the cleanse are carried out of the body and that all of your nutritional requirements are being met.

4. *Vegetables*

Vegetables are packed full of antioxidants, fiber, vitamins, minerals, and phytonutrients. We need at least six servings of vegetables a day to keep our bodies in a healthy, alkaline, and anabolic state. Incorporate cruciferous and colorful vegetables such as broccoli, kale, watercress, mustard greens, asparagus, peppers, sea vegetables, herbs and spices, etc. They help eliminate excess toxins and waste from the body and enhance beneficial bacteria populations. They reduce excess cholesterol and balance blood sugar levels. The only vegetable that should be avoided during the cleanse is white potatoes.

5. *Fruit*

Fruits contain bioflavonoids, antioxidants, phytonutrients, enzymes, vitamins, and minerals. Both the Canadian Food Guide and the U.S. Food Pyramid recommend a minimum of two servings of fresh fruit daily. Berries contain the highest amount of antioxidants, particularly blueberries, gogi berries, and acai berries. They help reduce inflammation, keep our blood vessels elastic, boost the immune system, and prevent cancer. Their natural enzymes are also beneficial for the digestive system.

6. *Lean Proteins*

Lean proteins help increase metabolic rate, regulate anabolic metabolism, and help maintain a proper blood sugar balance, which is crucial for fat loss. Protein contains amino acids, which are the raw materials responsible for regenerating the body. Lean proteins also increase thermogenesis, which is the body's ability to burn calories as heat.

7. *Water*

It is important to consume a minimum of eight 8-oz glasses of purified water daily. Next to oxygen, water is the most important nutrient we need to consume. It is essential for energy; it helps flush out toxins and waste products; it is responsible for regulating all our biological processes; it boosts our antiaging potential; and you can't live without it. The human body is 60–70 percent water.

Start your day off with a glass of purified water with a squeeze of lemon. This will help with the detoxification process and will hydrate your body.

8. *Flaxseeds*

Flaxseeds are high in omega-3 fatty acids, fiber, and lignans. Lignans are powerful anticancer compounds. They have antiviral, antibacterial, and antifungal properties. Flaxseeds are the preferred source of fiber because they contain both soluble and insoluble fibers, which act like a broom, sweeping up the toxins in the intestinal tract and keeping bowel movements regular. It is very important to have at least one bowel movement per day to ensure that waste and toxins are being eliminated. Daily consumption of flaxseeds will help balance blood sugar levels and contribute to fat loss.

In order to obtain all the nutrient benefits from flaxseeds, they need to be ground. The easiest way is to grind them in a coffee grinder. It takes seconds, and you can add it to your cereal, salads, or shakes. For convenience, I suggest grinding a week's worth at a time and storing them in a dark, sealed container in your fridge.

Supplements

Taking certain supplements will help support the detoxification process.

1. *Digestive Enzymes*

Digestive enzymes break down food into tiny particles that can be absorbed by the small intestine. They are important for proper liver function, cellular replication, and they give the digestive system support during detoxification.

2. *greens+ daily detox*

This excellent supplement aids in the gentle detoxification of the liver and gastrointestinal tract while providing antioxidant support.

3. *Probiotics*

Probiotics are beneficial bacteria that lower the levels of potentially toxic and cancerous chemicals inside the intestinal tract. These bacteria protect the intestinal lining to prevent toxins from being absorbed into your bloodstream. It is vital to have optimized bowel flora for detoxification.

PHASE ONE: SUMMARY

It is that simple. Eliminate those foods that are adding to your toxic load, and build a clean, seven-day diet consisting of delicious vegetables, whole grains, fruits, lean proteins, legumes, beans, water, and flaxseeds. Choose your favorite combinations and explore foods that you haven't tried yet. Make it fun! I am not forcing you into some crazy restricted diet. Quite the contrary, when you are hungry, eat! In fact, eat every couple of hours. Just be sure to eat from this list of great food choices and avoid those few items that I have clearly outlined for you.

Cleansing is an important starting point for any diet and it will prepare your body for a new way of eating. You now have the knowledge to create a successful seven-day cleanse, so set your goals and expect success. You can do it! Write down the following summary steps and post them on your refrigerator door for the duration of the first week of the Fat-Fighter Diet.

Foods to Eliminate
- all processed and refined foods
- dairy
- red meat
- white potatoes

Foods to Enjoy
- all fruits, especially berries
- all vegetables except white potatoes

- beans and legumes
- flaxseeds (ground)—1 tsp per day
- lean proteins—poultry, eggs, fish, tofu
- raw nuts and seeds
- water—minimum of eight glasses a day

Supplemental Support
- digestive enzymes—one capsule with each meal
- greens+ daily detox—one scoop a day
- probiotics—three capsules a day

7-DAY QUICK CLEANSE MEAL PLAN

To help you to get started right away I have included the following cleanse meal plan for you to follow. There are different amounts for men and women so please choose the category that is right for you.

Note: The female cleanse meal plan is approximately 1400 calories and the male cleanse meal plan is approximately 1800 calories. "F-Serving" = Female Serving / "M-Serving" = Male Serving.

Breakfast Options

Berrylicious Shake

Food Description	F-Serving	M-Serving	Recipe
Almond milk	½ cup	¾ cup	Mix banana, strawberries, blueberries, and almond milk, and blend. Add water if needed. Add ground flaxseeds and vanilla protein and blend an additional 10 seconds. Enjoy! Serves one.
Bananas	½	¾	
Blueberries	⅛ cup	⅛ cup	
Whey protein powder	3½ tbsp	4½ tbsp	
Flaxseed	3 tbsp	3½ tbsp	
Strawberries	⅛ cup	⅛ cup	

Oatmeal and Blueberries

Food Description	F-Serving	M-Serving	Recipe
Blueberries	⅓ cup	⅓ cup	In a pot, cook oatmeal in water on low heat, stirring continuously. Stir in vanilla extract and ground flaxseeds, making sure cereal is not too hot. Pour into bowl and stir in protein. Add fruit and serve. Enjoy! Serves one.
Oatmeal	⅓ cup	½ cup	
Whey protein powder	3 tbsp	4 tbsp	
Flaxseed	2 tbsp	3 tbsp	
Vanilla extract	⅓ tsp	⅓ tsp	
Filtered water	⅔ cup	1 cup	

Multi-Grain Cereal

Food Description	F-Serving	M-Serving	Recipe
Multi-Grain cereal	½ cup	¾ cup	Mix rice milk and cereal, then stir in protein. Add berries and ground flaxseeds. Enjoy! Serves one.
Whey protein powder	3 tbsp	5 tbsp	
Rice milk	½ cup	¾ cup	
Flaxseed	1 tbsp	3 tbsp	
Strawberries	5	5	

Egg White Omelet

Food Description	F-Serving	M-Serving	Recipe
Broccoli, raw (chopped)	½ cup	1 cup	In a bowl, combine egg whites. Lightly coat a non-stick pan with olive oil. Add vegetables and cook on medium heat until tender. Pour egg mixture on top. Reduce heat and cook for 5 minutes, flipping the omelet after five minutes. Enjoy! Serves one.
Egg whites	5	6	
Extra virgin olive oil	1 tbsp	1 tbsp	
Red peppers, sweet, chopped	½ cup	¾ cup	
Spinach, fresh	1 cup	1½ cup	
Cherry tomatoes	6	10	

Omega3 Omelet

Food Description	F-Serving	M-Serving	Recipe
Egg whites	2	3	In a bowl, combine eggs and egg whites. Lightly coat a nonstick pan with organic coconut oil. Add vegetables and cook on medium heat until tender. Pour egg mixture on top. Reduce heat and cook for 10 minutes, flipping the omelet after five minutes. Enjoy! Serves one.
omega 3 eggs	2	2	
Onions, sweet	¼	½	
Red peppers, chopped	¼ cup	½ cup	
Rice cheese, shredded	1 tbsp	4 tbsp	
Tomatoe, chopped or sliced	½	1	
Coconut oil	⅓ tbsp	⅔ tbsp	

Raspberry Soy Yogurt

Food Description	F-Serving	M-Serving	Recipe
Sunflower seeds	1 tsp	2 tbsp	Add sunflower seeds, protein, and raspberries to yogurt. Enjoy! Serves one.
Soy protein isolate	2 tbsp	2½ tbsp	
Soy yogurt	¾ cup	1 cup	
Raspberries	¼ cup	⅓ cup	

Blackberry Rice Shake

Food Description	F-Serving	M-Serving	Recipe
Blackberries	½ cup	½ cup	Place all ingredients, except protein powder, in blender. Blend until smooth. Add protein and blend for additional 10 seconds. Enjoy! Serves one.
Flaxseed oil	⅔ tbsp	1 tbsp	
Ice cubes	4	4	
Whey protein powder	4 tbsp	5 tbsp	
Vanilla extract	1 tsp	1 tsp	
Filtered water	⅓ cup	⅓ cup	
Rice milk	¾ cup	1 cup	

Lunch Options

Salmon Salad

Food Description	F-Serving	M-Serving	Recipe
Chives, chopped	3 tbsp	4 tbsp	On a large plate, mix peppers, radishes and green salad. Grill salmon and zucchini and place them on the salad. Sprinkle chives on top. Sprinkle lemon garlic dressing. Enjoy! Serves one. **Lemon Garlic Dressing:** olive oil, lemon, mustard, crushed garlic, and sea salt.
Dry mustard	1 tsp	1 tsp	
Extra virgin olive oil	1 tbsp	1½ tbsp	
Wild salmon	100 grams	115 grams	
Garlic	½ clove	¾ clove	
Lemon juice	6 tbsp	8 tbsp	
Mixed greens	2 cups	4 cups	
Red peppers	1 cup	1 cup	
Sea salt	½ tsp	½ tsp	
Zucchini, sliced	½ cup	1 cup	
Radishes	2	3	

Spinach Salad

Food Description	F-Serving	M-Serving	Recipe
Beets, grated	⅓ cup	½ cup	Remove the stems from the spinach and tear into bite-sized pieces. Mix spinach, grated beets, grated carrots, and sliced zucchini together. Boil egg and let cool. Then chop and add to mixture. Toss with lemon garlic dressing. Mix well and enjoy! Serves one. **Lemon Garlic Dressing:** olive oil, lemon, mustard, crushed garlic, and sea salt.
Carrots, grated	⅓ cup	½ cup	
Dry mustard	1 tsp	1 1/2 tsp	
Egg	2	3	
Extra virgin olive oil	1 tbsp	1 tbsp	
Garlic	½ clove	⅔ clove	
Lemon juice	4 tbsp	6 tbsp	
Sea salt	¼ tsp	¼ tsp	
Spinach	2 cups	2½ cups	
Zucchini, sliced	½ cup	¾ cup	

Turkey Sandwich

Food Description	F-Serving	M-Serving	Recipe
100% whole grain bread	2 slices	2 slices	Place turkey, tomato, carrots, cucumber, and soy mayonnaise on bread. Enjoy! Serves one.
Carrots, grated	2 tbsp	4 tbsp	
Cucumber	4 slices	4 slices	
Soy mayonnaise	¾ tbsp	1 tbsp	
Turkey breast meat	1 small	1 small	
Tomato	2 slices	4 slices	

Chicken Sandwich

Food Description	F-Serving	M-Serving	Recipe
Cucumber	4 slices	6 slices	Lightly toast bread (optional). Mix soy mayonnaise and onion together and spread over bread. Place chicken breast, lettuce, tomato, and cucumber on one slice of bread and cover with the other. Enjoy! Serves one.
Lettuce, shredded	¼ cup	¼ cup	
Green onions	½ tbsp	1 tbsp	
Soy mayonnaise	¾ tbsp	1 tbsp	
100% whole grain bread	2 slices	2 slices	
Tomato	3 slices	4 slices	
Chicken breast, grilled	½ cup	⅔ cup	

Tuna Salad

Food Description	F-Serving	M-Serving	Recipe
Alfalfa sprouts	¼ cup	¼ cup	In small bowl, mash chickpeas. Add soy mayonnaise, tuna, sprouts, mustard, and pepper, and mix well. This is wonderful in a pita or on bread with sprouts and some chopped tomato! Serves one.
100% whole grain bread	2 slices	2 slices	
Chickpeas, canned	¼ cup	⅓ cup	
Canned light tuna	3 ounces	4 ounces	
Dijon mustard	½ tsp	½ tsp	
Black pepper	½ tsp	½ tsp	
Tomatoes, chopped	⅓	½	
Soy mayonnaise	½ tbsp	1 tbsp	

Strawberry Pecan and Chicken Salad

Food Description	F-Serving	M-Serving	Recipe
Balsamic vinegar	2½ tbsp	3 tbsp	Mix salad greens and halved strawberries in a large salad bowl. Top with pecans, chicken, and vinaigrette. Serves one. **Vinaigrette:** in a small bowl, combine: sea salt, honey, dry mustard, onion, extra virgin olive oil and balsamic vinegar.
Dry mustard	½ tsp	¾ tsp	
Extra virgin olive oil	½ tbsp	1 tbsp	
Honey	1 tbsp	1 tbsp	
Mixed greens	1½ cups	2 cups	
Sea salt	⅓ tsp	½ tsp	
Onion powder	1 tsp	1 tsp	
Strawberries	8	10	
Pecans	5	5	
Chicken breast, grilled	½ cup	¾ cup	

Almond Stir Fry with Wild Rice

Food Description	F-Serving	M-Serving	Recipe
Bean sprouts	1/8 cup	1/8 cup	Chop all vegetables into small pieces. Lightly oil skillet with extra virgin olive oil. Over medium heat, cook all ingredients except rice. In a separate pot, cook rice according to instructions and serve together. Enjoy! Serves one.
Broccoli	1/8 cup	1/8 cup	
Extra virgin olive oil	1/3 tbsp	1/2 tbsp	
Garlic	1/4 clove	1/3 clove	
Ginger root	1/4 tsp	1/3 tsp	
Tofu, firm	4 slices	5 slices	
Almonds	6	8	
Onions	1/8 cup	1/8 cup	
Wild rice	1/8 cup	1/4 cup	
Sea salt	1/4 tsp	1/2 tsp	
Gluten-free tamari	1 tbsp	1 tbsp	

Dinner Options

Baked Salmon

Food Description	F-Serving	M-Serving	Recipe
Sea salt	⅓ tsp	⅓ tsp	Coat bottom of baking dish with olive oil; then layer the baking dish with onion, asparagus, and red pepper. Place salmon on vegetable bed in baking dish. Sprinkle salmon lightly with dill and garlic powder. Add water to baking dish and seal tightly with aluminum foil. Bake in preheated oven at 350°F for 35 minutes. Remove baking dish from oven and drain cooking liquid. Using spatula, scoop out vegetables with salmon and place on rice. Sprinkle with chives, black pepper, and sea salt, and serve. The asparagus will bleach out during cooking. If you prefer, it can be lightly steamed separately. Cook rice according to directions and serve with salmon and veggies. Enjoy! Serves one.
Asparagus	4 spears	4 spears	
Red pepper, chopped	¼ cup	¼ cup	
Chives, chopped	½ tsp	1 tsp	
Extra virgin olive oil	⅓ tbsp	½ tbsp	
Wild salmon	4 oz	5 oz	
Onions, sliced	¼ cup	¼ cup	
Long-grain brown rice	⅛ cup	¼ cup	
Dill weed, dried	¼ tsp	⅓ tsp	
Garlic powder	¼ tsp	⅓ tsp	
Black pepper	¼ tsp	⅓ tsp	

Chicken and Veggies

Food Description	F-Serving	M-Serving	Recipe
Asparagus	4 spears	6 spears	Steam and mash sweet potato, add olive oil and pumpkin seeds. Steam asparagus and Brussels sprouts. Bake chicken breast in oven at 350°F for 20 minutes or until done. Serve together. Enjoy! Serves one.
Brussels sprouts	4	5	
Chicken breast	1/3	1/2	
Extra virgin olive oil	1/2 tbsp	2/3 tbsp	
Pumpkin seeds	1/2 tbsp	1 tbsp	
Sweet potato	1 small	1 small	

Ahi Tuna and Arugula Salad

Food Description	F-Serving	M-Serving	Recipe
Ahi Tuna, boneless (premium)	4 ounces	6 ounces	**Dressing:** Combine lemon and lime juice together with shallot in a bowl, and season with black pepper and sea salt. Combine with olive oil and mix together. **Salad:** In another bowl, combine tuna, cherry tomatoes, avocado, and toasted pine nuts. Add arugula, and gently toss with other ingredients. Add dressing and finish seasoning to taste. Enjoy! Serves one.
Arugula	2½ cups	5	
Avocado, sliced	⅛ cup	½ cup	
Extra virgin olive oil	½ tbsp	⅔ tbsp	
Lemon juice, fresh squeezed	1	1	
Lime juice, fresh squeezed	½	½	
Pine nuts	6	7	
Sea salt	¼ tsp	¼ tsp	
Shallots, chopped	6 tbsp	6 tbsp	
Black pepper	⅓ tsp	⅓ tsp	
Cherry tomatoes	6	8	

Veggie Pasta

Food Description	F-Serving	M-Serving	Recipe
Bean sprouts	⅛ cup	⅛ cup	Soak texturized vegetable protein (TVP) for 10 minutes in water. Boil pasta for 7–10 minutes. Chop all vegetables and stir fry with TVP and olive oil for 3 minutes. Mix with strained pasta. Add organic pasta sauce on top. Enjoy! Serves one.
Broccoli, chopped	¼ cup	¼ cup	
Brown rice pasta	½ cup	⅔ cup	
Celery, chopped	⅛ cup	⅛ cup	
Extra virgin olive oil	1 tbsp	1 tbsp	
Yellow peppers, chopped	¼	¼	
Texturized vegetable protein	¾ cup	1 cup	
Organic tomato sauce	¼ cup	¼ cup	

Vegetable Shrimp Stir-Fry

Food Description	F-Serving	M-Serving	Recipe
Celery, chopped	2 stalks	3 stalks	In nonstick sauté pan, add oil, onion, pepper, celery, and garlic. Cook until vegetables are tender; then add shrimp, tomato puree, water, celery salt, thyme, and black pepper. Bring mixture to a boil; then simmer for 5–10 minutes. Enjoy! Serves one.
Shrimp	15	19	
Extra virgin olive oil	⅔ tbsp	1 tbsp	
Garlic	1 clove	1 clove	
Onions, sliced	⅔ cup	1 cup	
Red peppers, chopped	¾ cup	¾ cup	
Sea salt	¼ tsp	¼ tsp	
Black pepper	¼ tsp	¼ tsp	
Thyme, dried	½ tsp	½ tsp	
Tomato puree	1 cup	1 cup	

Chicken a la Skew

Food Description	F-Serving	M-Serving	Recipe
Celery, sliced	1 stalk	1 stalk	Cook rice as per package instructions. Cut chicken and vegetables into bite-sized chunks. Thread on skewer. Broil for 20 minutes, turning several times. With the leftover oil, baste a couple of times. Serve with rice. Enjoy! Serves one.
Chicken breast, bone and skin removed	½	⅔	
Extra virgin olive oil	⅔ tbsp	1 tbsp	
Mushroom, sliced	1	1	
Onions, sliced	¼	¼	
Red peppers, chopped	¼	¼	
Long-grain brown rice	¼ cup	¼ cup	
Zucchini, sliced	¼	¼	

Grilled Calamari on Greens

Food Description	F-Serving	M-Serving	Recipe
Balsamic vinegar	2 tbsp	3 tbsp	Grill calamari in oil; then add sliced red pepper and zucchini and grill another 5–7 minutes. Place on mixed salad greens, top with oil, balsamic vinegar, and crushed garlic. Enjoy! Serves one.
Calamari	5 oz.	6 oz.	
Extra virgin olive oil	1 tbsp	1½ tbsp	
Garlic	1 clove	1 clove	
Mixed greens	1½ cups	2 cups	
Red peppers	½	¾	
Zucchini	½	¾	

Snack Options

Abundant Energy Elixir

Food Description	F-Serving	M-Serving	Recipe
Bananas	1/2 small	1/2 medium	Place all ingredients except almonds in a blender and blend at high speed for about 35 seconds until smooth. Enjoy the nuts on the side. Serves one.
Ice cubes	3	4	
Almonds	10	13	
Whey protein powder	3 tbsp	3 tbsp	
Strawberries	4	6	
Filtered water	1 1/2 cup	1 1/2 cup	

Almond Butter Crackers

Food Description	F-Serving	M-Serving	Recipe
Brown rice crackers	2	3	Spread almond butter on brown rice crackers. Enjoy with a protein shake. Serves one.
Almond butter	½ tbsp	⅔ tbsp	
Whey protein powder	2 tbsp	3 tbsp	
Filtered water	1 cup	1 cup	

Apple and Nuts

Food Description	F-Serving	M-Serving	Recipe
Apples	½	⅔	Eat soy nuts and fruit. Serves one.
Soy nuts	¼ cup	⅓ cup	

Veggie Crackers and Cheese

Food Description	F-Serving	M-Serving	Recipe
Red pepper	⅓	⅓	Slice red pepper and cheese and place on crackers. Enjoy! Serves one.
Brown rice crackers	2	3	
Rice cheese	2 oz.	3 oz.	

Hummus and Veggies

Food Description	F-Serving	M-Serving	Recipe
Hummus	1 tbsp	1 tbsp	Dip veggies and cheese into hummus, and enjoy. Serves one.
Red pepper	½	⅓	
Soy cheese	3 slices	3⅓ slices	
Broccoli	4 flowerets	4 flowerets	
Cauliflower	4 flowerets	4 flowerets	

Tasty Celery and Nuts

Food Description	F-Serving	M-Serving	Recipe
Celery	3½ stalks	4 stalks	Spread almond butter on celery stalk. Eat with soy nuts. Enjoy! Serves one.
Almond butter	1 tbsp	1 tbsp	
Soy nuts	15	20	

Berry Blast Shake

Food Description	F-Serving	M-Serving	Recipe
Blackberries	⅓ cup	½ cup	Place all ingredients except protein powder in blender. Blend until smooth. Add protein and blend for an additional 10 seconds. Serves one.
Blueberries	⅓ cup	½ cup	
Flaxseed oil	⅓ tbsp	½ tbsp	
Ice cubes	3	3	
Soy or whey protein isolate	2 tbsp	2 tbsp	
Strawberries	3	4	
Filtered water	1½ cups	1½ cups	

Watermelon and Soy

Food Description	F-Serving	M-Serving	Recipe
Soy nuts	¼ cup	⅓ cup	Eat fresh and enjoy! Serves one.
Watermelon	⅓ wedge	½ wedge	

Healthy Fat Trail Mix

Food Description	F-Serving	M-Serving	Recipe
Gogi berries	15	20	Eat raw nuts, seeds, and berries together. Enjoy! Serves one.
Almonds	6	10	
Pumpkin seeds	10	15	
Soy nuts	10	15	

ACTION

Complete Phase One by cleansing both your body and your kitchen. Doing so will prime your system for the results to come from Phase Two.

PHASE TWO: PROPEL

Now that you have completed Phase One of the Fat-Fighter Diet, you are ready to move on to Phase Two in which you will learn exactly how much, how often, when, and what you should be eating. The Fat-Fighter Diet is designed to be a sustainable program that you can follow for the rest of your life. Since the diet will change as your body changes, you will be able to adjust your portions according to your body composition and goals at any given time. There are many fabulous foods to choose from, allowing for flexibility and achievable results.

PROPEL: HOW MUCH?

In today's supersized world, the sheer volume of food that people are consuming is the most significant contributor to obesity. According to the National Heart, Lung, and Blood Institute, North American portion sizes have expanded along with our waistlines, and our perception of what constitutes an appropriate portion has become wildly distorted. Many studies have documented that the more food that is put in front of us, the more we eat.

It is important to note that even if the food being consumed is healthy organic fruits, vegetables, lean proteins, and essential fats, too much of anything can contribute to fat gain. That said, I have yet to meet one person with a weight problem whose sole source of calories were from the above-mentioned items. This is likely because healthy foods promote hormonal balance and create a lasting sense of satiation—food cravings diminish and appetite balance is restored. For the most part, people are eating too much food because they are eating the wrong foods.

WHAT ABOUT CALORIES?

Do you know how many calories you are eating each day? No one wants to spend time calorie counting, but it is an excellent exercise to add up your daily calorie intake for a week or 10 days. Once you get a sense of how many calories you are consuming now, followed by what it looks and feels like to be eating the correct number of calories daily, it will become second nature. If you need help discovering how many calories are in certain foods, you can visit www.ebodi.com or check out the free calorie counter at the U.S.D.A. Web site (www.usda.gov).

A calorie is defined as a measure of heat energy. When a food is heated, it releases a certain amount of energy. The more calories there are in a food, the more heat energy is released. Calories are also related to the fat that you have stored on your body. Body fat is basically stored energy (calories) just waiting to be burned. Certain activities, such as competing in a marathon, burn a lot more calories than, say, gardening. Our bodies are incredibly good at storing fat and, as explained previously, become increasingly more so each time you participate in a low-calorie diet. To lose body fat, you must create a calorie deficit, which is done by reducing calorie intake, increasing calorie expenditure, or by doing a combination of both. However, as you know, cutting calories alone is not a guaranteed path to fat loss. Many people think that weight loss can be boiled down to a simple equation.

True of False?

Consume less calories than you burn = weight loss
Consume more calories than you burn = weight gain

The problem with this equation is that there is no differentiation between fat loss and a reduction in muscle or water weight. This pertains only to the number on the scale. Please recall what I said previously about building materials needed for this new body you are building: The *quality* of calories is as important as the *quantity* of calories. The human body is *not* a laboratory calorimeter. There is more to the equation than simply calories in minus calories out. As with all things, the physics law of "Every action has an equal and opposite reaction" applies. The action of eating foods imparts a reaction of hormonal response in the body.

Two thousand calories per day of refined sugars and hydrogenated oils will produce vastly different results, both esthetically and in terms of your health, compared to 2,000 calories per day of complex carbohydrates, lean proteins, and essential fatty acids.

How Many Calories Are Right for Burning Fat, Increasing Muscle, or Improving Health?

This chapter will walk you through your individualized equations so that you will know exactly how many calories you need to consume in order to meet your goals. This is valuable information! For those of you who are less mathematically inclined, use the general guidelines below, or go to the wellness guidance system www.ebodi.com, where all the calculating is done for you. You can also use the free wellness analysis to calculate your body fat percentage.

General Caloric guidelines

Fat Loss
Women: 1,400–1,800 calories per day
Men: 2,200–2,600 calories per day

Healthy Lifestyle
Women: 1,900–2,100 calories per day
Men: 2,700–3,000 calories per day

Increase Lean Muscle and Strength
Women: 2,200–2,500 calories per day
Men: 3,100–4,000 calories per day

Personalized Caloric Guide

Whether your goal is to lose fat, increase lean muscle and strength, or to develop and maintain a healthy lifestyle, determining the correct number of calories your body needs is vital to your success. The number of calories your body needs each day is called your total daily energy expenditure or TDEE.

In order to properly calculate your TDEE, you will need to do some math (nothing fancy, I promise). We are going to use a formula invented by American exercise physiologists Frank Katch and William McArdle. This formula takes into account a person's body fat percentage, activity level, and base metabolic rate in order to determine that person's specific daily expenditure.

Step One:
Calculate your base metabolic rate or BMR as follows:
BMR = 370 + (21.6 × lean body mass in kilograms)

For example, let's say you are a woman weighing 150 lbs with 30 percent body fat.

Weight = 150 lbs (or 68 kg)
Body fat is 30 percent (or 45 lbs of fat)
Lean body mass = 105 lbs or 47.7 kg
BMR = 370 + (21.6 × 47.7) = 1,400 calories

This means that even if you stayed in bed all day, you would burn 1,400 calories.

Step Two:
Your activity level is the second component of your metabolism. In order to find your TDEE, simply multiply your BMR by your activity factor:

Sedentary: You currently do little or no exercise (BMR × 1.2)

Lightly active: You do light exercise/sports one to three days per week (BMR × 1.375)

Moderately active: You do moderate exercise/sports three to five days per week (BMR × 1.55)

Very active: You do hard exercise/sports six or seven days per week (BMR × 1.725)

Extremely active: You do hard daily exercise/sports and a physical job or twice daily training, i.e., marathon, contest, etc. (BMR × 1.9)

For example, if your BMR is 1,400 calories and you are lightly active (activity factor 1.375), your TDEE is 1,400 × 1.375 or 1,925 calories per day. This is the amount of calories you should be consuming each day based upon your weight, percent body fat, and activity level.

Adjusting Your Calories for Your Goal
The final step in determining the precise amount of food you should consume is to factor in your goal. Different goals require different amounts of calories. Adjust your TDEE according to the following goals.

Fat Loss

Take your TDEE and subtract 20 percent. This is the perfect amount of calorie deficit for fat loss; any more could cause a loss of muscle. For example, if your TDEE is 1,925 calories per day, multiply 1,925 × .20. This equals 385. Subtract 385 from 1,925 (1,925 – 385) = 1,540 calories per day.

Important Fat Loss Note: Because of the body's starvation response, it is important to remain at the 20 percent reduced calorie level for no more than five days at a time. Be sure to return to your TDEE caloric level once per week. This will trick your body into increasing its metabolic rate and prevent slowing of your metabolism. An easy way to do this is to have a "reward meal" every five days. This is a great place to put that piece of pizza you have been craving and will allow for a slight increase in calories for that day.

Healthy Lifestyle

When your goal is to develop and maintain a healthy lifestyle, the TDEE is the perfect amount of calories you should consume. Just be sure to monitor your *activity level* and adjust your calories accordingly. One simple rule of thumb I tell all of my clients is to *eat less when you do less.* This will ensure that your caloric intake does not exceed your caloric output.

Increase Lean Muscle and Strength

When you are trying to increase the amount of lean muscle tissue you have, it is important that your caloric intake supports this goal. To calculate the right amount of calories for you, take your TDEE and add 20 percent. For example, if your TDEE is 1,925 calories per day, multiply 1,925 × 1.20. This equals 2,310 calories per day. These extra calories will ensure that you are consuming enough calories and nutrients to support your muscle- and strength-building goal.

ACTION

Determine how many calories are right for you. Be sure to recalculate this number every four to six weeks to account for changes in your body composition. Remember that as your fat-to-muscle ratio changes, your calorie requirements may actually increase due to an increase in lean muscle tissue.

PROPEL: HOW OFTEN?

Changing your meal frequency will afford you the most bang for your buck when it comes to improving your nutrition program. The simple act of adding two small snacks between your three main meals (breakfast, lunch, and dinner) will speed up most metabolisms to the point where body fat is quickly and noticeably reduced. This is one of the most important components that you must understand and for those who like to eat, one of the most enjoyable. When combined with resistance training, this effect is multiplied due to the increase in muscle mass and concurrent rise in the metabolic rate. I often compare the relationship of food and metabolism to that of fire and wood; when good-quality wood is added in the right amounts at regular intervals, the fire burns hotter and hotter. The same principle applies to your metabolism—the right foods at the right times will cause your metabolism to burn white hot!

Many of my clients will express their concern over eating every three hours. "I do not have the time" is perhaps the number one reason given for not doing so. Remember that we are not talking about five full-sized meals here. Rather, we are talking about three regular meals and two snacks. These snacks can be very fast to prepare and consume. For example, a palm-sized portion of raw nuts and seeds with an apple, or cottage cheese and fruit would both fit the bill and neither would take long to prepare. The goal with your snacks (as with all your meals) is to make sure it consists of a protein, fat, and carbohydrate food source. If you are unsure as to what type of protein, carbohydrate, or fat to eat, don't worry—read on and you will discover everything you need to know! You can also opt for a protein shake or meal replacement. Just try to avoid artificial sweeteners, trans fats, and fillers. Planning, scheduling, and preparing your meals in advance is absolutely vital to your success.

Benefits of Increasing Meal Frequency

The benefits of eating five to six small, nutrient-packed meals per day far outweigh any inconvenience posed by their preparation. These benefits include:

1. *Increased metabolism:* Frequent, small feedings stoke the fire of your metabolism.

2. *Increased energy:* Small amounts of complex carbohydrates, proteins, and fats throughout the day will increase energy levels. In addition, digesting a smaller meal requires less energy than digesting a large meal, which leaves you with more energy.

3. *Increased digestion and assimilation:* When you eat small meals more frequently, the body is better able to digest and assimilate the nutrients ingested.

4. *Decreased cravings:* Skipping meals causes blood sugar to fall, resulting in vicious food cravings. Persistent blood sugar fluctuations can lead to type 2 diabetes, obesity, heart disease, and stroke. Frequent feeding will balance your blood sugar levels, keeping cravings at bay.

5. *Increased lean muscle growth:* Eating protein at regular intervals allows for a steady flow of amino acids to your muscle cells where they can be used to promote new tissue growth. This steady flow of amino acids is also important in the fight against muscle wasting or catabolism, which often occurs with other diets.

6. *Improved cholesterol profiles:* A study published in the British Medical Journal found that of more than 14,600 men and women aged 45–75, total cholesterol and LDL counts declined as meal frequency increased. Participants who ate five or six times a day had the lowest total cholesterol and LDL, while those who ate one or two large meals a day had the highest measurements.

Never Skip Meals

No matter what your goal, skipping meals is to be avoided at all costs. This is the most common mistake people make when trying to improve their physical appearance and overall health. Skipping meals will result in a slower metabolism, muscle loss, and low energy. The most commonly skipped meal is breakfast. Many people feel they just do not have the time. To these people I suggest planning ahead—remember, success is planned while failure never is—and getting up 15 minutes earlier. (It takes only a few minutes to prepare oatmeal and a protein shake, for example). Because you have not eaten since eight o'clock the previous evening, when you skip breakfast you are essentially fasting for more than half a day, which is long enough to trick your body into a famine response and slow your metabolism (the word "breakfast" means "a break from fasting"). As paradoxical as it sounds, eating nutrient-packed meals more frequently will cause you to *lose* fat, while eating less frequently will cause you to *gain* fat!

Frequent Eating Made Easy

Eating three meals and two snacks each day is really simple if you use the following tips:

1. Buy a portable cooler and keep it in the car and/or at work. Leave your meals and snacks in the cooler to keep them handy and fresh.
2. Leave healthy snack items at work for you to enjoy.
3. Never leave home without water.
4. Stash some protein bars in your purse, pocket, and the glove compartment of your car.
5. Purchase good-quality resealable containers to store your food in.

ACTION
Plan ahead. Prepare yourself for eating three meals and two snacks each day.

PROPEL: WHEN?

I know what you are thinking—eat when you are hungry, right? Wrong. The sensation of hunger is often dehydration in disguise and by the time you are feeling hungry, your blood sugar is already taking a downward turn, leading to feelings of irritability and lethargy. Whether your goal is to increase lean muscle and strength, to lose fat, or to improve overall health, you must schedule your meals ahead of time. The key points to remember when it comes to timing your meals are as follows.

1. *Eat your first meal as early in the day as possible.* By doing so you are kick-starting your metabolic rate early in the day. You will also find it much easier to have three meals and two snacks if your first meal is in the early morning.

2. *Eat every two and a half to three hours.* Eating small, nutrient-dense, and low-calorie meals throughout the day is the fastest way to boost metabolism while improving nutrient assimilation and fat burning.

3. *Eat the majority of your calories before late afternoon.* This is where the North American lifestyle goes astray. Most North Americans typically eat very little in the morning and have their largest meal of the day at night. This does little

for improving metabolism and maintaining lean muscle tissue. A much healthier option is to make lunch the principal meal of the day, which allows for these calories to be burned while doing the day's activities.

4. *Consume a post-workout protein and carbohydrate drink.* Within 30 minutes of finishing your resistance-training workout, consume a protein and carbohydrate beverage. This post-workout drink should contain:
   - Between 50–100 g of carbohydrate
   - Between 25–40 g of protein
   - 5 g of creatine monohydrate

Doing so will help speed recovery, replenish depleted glycogen stores, reduce cortisol levels, and restore energy. Please see Chapter 13 for some great shake recipes!

5. *Reduce calories as the day progresses.* Gradually reducing calories throughout the day is known as caloric tapering. This is a technique that is often used by athletes who wish to become lean and reduce body fat. Eating less as the day progresses ensures that you will be eating the fewest amount of calories before you sleep, which is the time when your metabolism is at its slowest.

6. *Do not eat after 8 p.m.* Eating after 8 p.m. can interfere with the body's production of melatonin, a powerful cancer-fighting, antiaging hormone. In order to get the most from your sleep, schedule your last meal two to three hours before bed. If you must eat after eight (as part of your regular schedule), make sure it is a low-calorie protein source such as low-fat organic cottage cheese or a whey protein-based drink. Be sure to keep the calories (and carbohydrates) low for any meals eaten after 8 p.m. and, as always, be sure to avoid sugary foods!

ACTION
Schedule each of your meals and snacks into your day planner. Time each of your meals for optimum results.

PROPEL: WHAT?

Now that I have convinced you of the importance of frequent eating, it is time to discuss just what these meals are to be comprised of. With the Fat Fighter Diet, it is important that every meal accomplish certain goals:

1. Each meal must promote optimal health.
2. Each meal must support and promote a healthy metabolism.
3. Each meal must help to stabilize blood sugar levels.

In order to accomplish the above three goals, each of your meals must contain protein, carbohydrate, and fat in the right ratios. There are no gimmicks here. Eating the correct quantity and balance of protein, carbohydrates, and fats together in the same meal will produce better results than eating them separately. Let's take a quick look at each of these macronutrients on their own. Afterwards, we will look at how we should combine them to create your perfect plate.

Protein

Protein is so important that when the Greeks named it, they called it *protos*, which means "to come first." Of the "big three" macronutrients, only protein has the unique distinction of being directly responsible for building, repairing, and maintaining muscle tissue. Muscle tissue, as you now know, is absolutely essential for optimizing metabolism and improving body composition. Proteins are made up of some or all of the possible 20 amino acids. The body cannot use the protein you eat unless all 20 of the necessary amino acids are present. Our bodies are quite remarkable. We are able to produce 11 amino acids naturally; however, the remaining nine *essential amino acids* must be obtained from the foods that we eat.

The Fat-Fighter Diet's Approved Protein Foods (Phase Two)
The following is a list of proteins you can choose from in Phase Two:

- Chicken: Free-range, organic, grain-fed
- Extra-lean red meat: Organic beef, buffalo, and venison (Please limit consumption of red meat to a maximum of once per week.)
- Fish: Wild salmon, canned light tuna (in water), haddock, pickerel, herring sardines, crab, halibut, mackerel, and tilapia
- Nuts and seeds

- Organic dairy: Low-fat cottage cheese, milk, yogurt, and kefir
- Organic eggs: One yolk for every six eggs
- Protein isolates: Whey, soy, and hemp
- Sea vegetables
- Shellfish: Shrimp, scallops, and lobster
- Tempeh
- Tofu
- Turkey: Free-range, organic, grain-fed

Biological Value of Proteins

The biological value of protein is a ranking system that represents the efficiency with which a protein is utilized by the body for tissue growth (anabolism). The higher the biological value, the greater the absorption and uptake by the body.

Protein Biological Value

- High alpha whey isolates 159
- Whey protein isolates 110–159
- Whey protein concentrates 104
- Whole eggs 100
- Cow's milk 91
- Egg whites 88
- Fish 83
- Beef 80
- Chicken 79
- Milk protein 77
- Tofu/Tempeh 74
- Rice 59
- Nuts and seeds 49
- Legumes 49
- Sea vegetables 49

Vary Your Proteins

Because of the differences in biological values and amino acid profiles, it is important to vary your protein choices. Try combining different types of protein foods together in the same meal and vary your proteins throughout the week.

Protein and Fat Loss

When it comes to losing body fat, protein is king. Protein has the highest fat-burning effect of all macronutrients. When you eat, a certain amount of calories are burned because of the energy required to digest the food. This is known as the thermic effect of food. When you eat protein, as much as 30 percent of the calories are used up digesting the protein. If you were to eat 100 calories worth of protein, 30 calories would be used up by the digestion process alone, leaving only 70 calories for your body to contend with. This thermic effect is a major ally for you if you are waging war against body fat. In addition to protein, you are about to discover what great allies complex carbohydrates and essential fatty acids are as well. To take full advantage of this thermic effect, eat approximately 30 percent of your daily calories as protein.

Eat Protein with Each Meal

Be prepared. When confronted with less than optimal options, make sure you have some protein on hand. This is easier to do than it sounds. Simply fill a shaker bottle (you can find them at your supermarket) with two scoops of protein powder and leave it in the car and at the office. At three o'clock, just add water and enjoy! While this is second choice to a whole food meal consisting of protein, complex carbohydrates, and essential fatty acids, it is far superior to junk food or not eating at all.

Eating protein at regular intervals throughout the day is important for five reasons:

1. Protein, unlike carbohydrates and fats, cannot be stored by the body for future use. Therefore we must be sure to ingest adequate amounts throughout the day.
2. Protein foods are beneficial in reducing hunger and cravings. In a 2003 study published in the *Current Opinion in Clinical Nutrition and Metabolic Care*, consuming protein was shown to be more satiating (the feeling of being full or satisfied) than both carbohydrates and fats.
3. If you do not get enough protein in a given day, the body will become catabolic and break down muscle tissue to satisfy requirements (also known as muscle wasting).
4. Protein helps to stimulate the release of the hormone glucagon. This helps to regulate the hormone insulin, which is important for reducing adult onset diabetes (type 2) and obesity. Glucagon also stimulates the use of

fat for energy and helps shift the metabolism into burning mode instead of storing mode.

5. Protein is essential to the building and maintenance of your body's greatest metabolic asset, your muscles.

Protein is a nutrient we just can't live without. Give it the respect it deserves by making it a priority with every meal. Your muscles and metabolism will thank you.

Carbohydrates

Of all the macronutrients, carbohydrates are the most misunderstood. Many diets capitalize on this confusion, touting the benefits of no-carb, low-carb, and slow-carb. No wonder people are so confused! Before we decide all carbohydrates are bad, let's take a closer look at what they are and what they do.

Carbohydrates are not just breads and pasta. Carbohydrates include everything from refined sugar to vegetables to whole-wheat bread to an apple. All of these foods fall under the term "carbohydrate," which is a major reason for all the confusion.

During digestion, carbohydrates are broken down into glucose, the preferred source of energy for the body. Carbohydrates can also be stored inside your muscles as glycogen for future use. Carbohydrates play a vital role in the energy systems of the body, and they contain many crucial vitamins and minerals. Never completely eliminate carbohydrate foods from your diet.

Carbohydrates also have a "protein-sparing" effect. When you eat carbohydrates with protein, the protein is spared from being used for energy and can be left to do the important job of building lean muscle tissue.

The Fat-Fighter Diet's Approved Carbohydrates (Phase Two)

The following is a list of approved carbohydrates you can choose from:

- Complex: 100 percent whole grains, brown rice, beans, legumes, lentils, sweet potatoes, carrots, oatmeal, bran, and barley
- Fibrous: Vegetables such as green beans, spinach, kale, asparagus, peas, collard greens, mushrooms, broccoli, lettuce, peppers, and cauliflower
- Simple: All fruits, such as blueberries, raspberries, apples, strawberries, plums, bananas, grapes, grapefruit, oranges, peaches, pears, and nectarines

Sugar: Public Enemy No. 1

Regardless of your fitness goal, sugar is the one carbohydrate you should avoid at all costs. Fat-free does not mean sugar-free, and in many cases sugar is just as bad (or worse) than certain fats! Sugar is the contributing factor in many health-related problems, including all of the following:

- Acceleration of cancers
- Acceleration of the aging process
- Decreased HDL or "good" cholesterol
- Depletion of minerals from the body
- Diabetes
- Elevated levels of acidity in the body
- Hypoglycemia
- Increased LDL or "bad" cholesterol
- Obesity
- Suppression of immune system

When you are trying to improve your body and health, steering clear of sugar is a great place to start. Be sure to read all labels and look for any hidden sugars and artificial sweeteners. Be aware that any ingredient ending in *-ose* is a sugar. If sugar is listed in the first few ingredients, select another product. A good alternative to sugar is stevia, which is a natural herb that is sweeter than sugar, but does not impact blood sugar levels. By cutting back on sugar, you will see improvements not just in fat loss but in your mood and health as well.

How Much Is Enough?

The debate over how many carbohydrates one should consume as a percentage of total calories has gone on for years. The fact is that of the three types of carbohydrate foods listed above, there are some that should be eaten more frequently and in greater amounts than others. The reason for this lies in the way our bodies react to certain foods when we eat them. When it comes to carbohydrates, the speed at which they are digested and turned into glucose (sugar) in your bloodstream is important. Once eaten, certain carbohydrates will digest very quickly, causing a sudden and rapid rise in our blood sugar levels. When this happens, the pancreas secretes insulin to balance out the rising blood sugar. The problem with this is fourfold:

1. When blood sugar and insulin levels are up, the body shuts down lipolysis or the release of fat for energy.
2. Chronic elevations in insulin can lead to hypoglycemia and type 2 diabetes.
3. High blood sugar levels and the resulting high insulin levels cause lipogenesis. Lipogenesis is the storage of fat ("lipo" means fat and "genesis" means formation).
4. High blood sugar levels and the resulting insulin response will also accelerate the aging process through a process called glycation. This occurs when proteins react with sugars, impairing the protein's function.

The human body is programmed to store fat. Our ancestors endured periods of feast and famine, and our bodies learned to adapt by storing fat to be used for energy during times of famine. Insulin is a storage hormone that is called into action every time you eat, especially when you eat or drink carbohydrates that elicit a rapid rise in blood sugar. Insulin drives the sugar (as well as protein and fat) from our blood into our cells to be stored as fat for later use. In order to avoid a sudden and rapid rise in blood sugar and the resulting insulin response, your carbohydrate foods should be primarily fibrous and complex together with *some* fruit.

The Glycemic Index

Any discussion on carbohydrates is not complete without talking about the glycemic index of foods. The glycemic index is a system of ranking various foods based on their immediate effect on blood sugar levels. The glycemic index measures how much your blood sugar increases over a period of two or three hours after a meal. When choosing carbohydrate foods, it is best to choose foods that are either low- or moderate-glycemic. High-glycemic foods should be eaten very sparingly. Even when combined with a protein or fat (which will, in effect, slow the digestion of the high-glycemic food), the low nutritive value of most high-glycemic foods is reason enough to avoid them.

The higher the number, the greater the blood sugar response. A low GI food will cause a small rise, while a high GI food will trigger a dramatic spike.

Glucose is given a value of 100 and other carbohydrates are given a number relative to glucose.

Glycemic Index Range
Low GI = 55 or less
Medium GI = 56–65
High GI = 65 or more

High-Glycemic Foods		Medium-Glycemic Foods		Low-Glycemic Foods	
French bread	100	banana	60	brown rice	55
glucose	100	beets	60	slow-cook oatmeal	55
rice cake	100	brown sugar	60	wild rice	55
milk chocolate	95	honey (unpasteurized)	60	apple juice	50
baked potato	93	pineapple	60	sweet potato	50
white rice	85	raw carrots	60	orange	40
corn flakes	83	watermelon	60	whole-wheat pasta	40
corn	80	white pasta	60	apple	36
french fries	80	white rice	60	pear	36
ice cream	80	(ripe) banana	56	skim milk	32
pretzels	80	barley malt	56	green beans	30
honey (pasteurized)	75	maple syrup	56	lentils	30
table sugar	75	pita bread	56	kidney beans	27
white flour	75	barley malt	56	barley	25
Cheerios	74	popcorn	56	grapefruit	25
graham crackers	74			fructose (avoid)	20
cooked carrots	71			rice bran	18
raisins	70-95			greens+	10
white bread/bagel	70-72			spices	10-20
				stevia	0

Sources:
Dr. Vincent Demarco, The Clinic for Optimal Health and Rejuvenation.
Sam Graci, *The Food Connection* (Toronto: Macmillan Canada, 2001), p. 172.

Lower the Glycemic Index of Any Meal

Sometimes we encounter situations where food choices are not optimal and we have to eat high-glycemic foods. In those instances, try the following:

1. *Add fiber:* Sprinkle food with flaxseed, bran, and wheat germ. Fiber slows the absorption of sugar. You should consume a minimum of 30 g of fiber per day, but most North Americans eat less than half that amount. Fiber has been shown to improve digestion, eliminate constipation, lower cholesterol levels, increase satiety and, of course, balance blood sugar levels. A Harvard Medical School study found that women who consumed the least amount of fiber were 31 percent more likely to be diagnosed with diabetes. For some people, using a dietary fiber supplement is an easy and convenient way of ensuring adequate consumption of this important nutrient.

2. *Add "good fat":* Flaxseed oil, flaxseeds, omega-3 fish oil, walnut oil, extra-virgin olive oil, pumpkinseed oil, and canola oil are healthy fats that will slow the absorption of the food, thus slowing the rise in blood sugar.

3. *Add protein:* The addition of a protein food source will also slow the digestion of the higher glycemic foods.

4. *Add acid:* Acidic food will slow the absorption of sugar. Good choices would include lemon juice, apple cider vinegar, and red wine vinegar.

Carbohydrate Key Points

Remember to stick to the following guidelines and you will master the carbohydrate confusion once and for all:

1. Consume more fibrous carbohydrates (especially vegetables) with every meal. Each of your meals should include approximately 40 percent of its calories as carbohydrates.
2. Choose complex carbohydrates (whole grains, brown rice, sweet potatoes, oatmeal, barley, spelt, and kamut).
3. Consume *some* simple carbohydrates (fruits).
4. Avoid commercial carbohydrate foods (chips, crackers, cookies).
5. Avoid refined sugar and foods that contain refined sugar (bars, candy).

For most people, following the previous rules will produce fantastic results. However, for a small percentage of the population, further tweaking is required. For those who wish to take their fat loss progress to the next level, I suggest timing their carbohydrate intake to coincide with the post-workout adaptation window. This means eating fewer carbohydrates in your last meal of the day and more carbohydrates immediately after your resistance-training workout. This is the time when your body needs them most and when they are least likely to be stored as fat. One simple way of doing this is to remove carbohydrates (except vegetables) from your last meal of the day and add those carbs to your post-workout meal. This will leave vegetables, fats, and protein in your evening meal and will work to further lower both calories and blood sugar in the evening.

Eliminating carbohydrates is the wrong way to approach your diet and fitness program. Learn to choose your carbohydrate foods more carefully, while focusing on quality as well as quantity. Be sure to consume natural source carbohydrates as opposed to those that are refined and manufactured. Eat smaller amounts of those carbohydrate foods that are higher in sugar and calories (such as white potato, white rice, and white pasta) and more of those that are higher in nutrients (such as greens, whole-grain breads, sea vegetables, berries, spinach, and broccoli). Doing so will give you a lifetime of health, fitness, and fat loss.

Fats

The word "fat" can still send a chill through the heart of even the most seasoned aerobics junkie. I can recall when "fat phobia" was at its height. It was the early 1980s and I was watching an infomercial featuring a well-known (at the time) weight-loss "expert" peddle her wares on late-night television. This woman (who will remain anonymous) wheeled a huge wagon of fat onto the stage while screaming "Fat makes you fat" over and over again. The whole country believed this and set out to remove all fat from their diets. All of a sudden "fat-free" this and "fat-free" that were everywhere. People took to this fad like crazy, consuming fat-free ice cream, fat-free cookies, fat-free *everything*! It seemed like we finally had the answer—and it was so obvious—fat makes you fat!

How wrong we were. Shortly we started to see a rapid increase in obesity. Diabetes was up too. In addition, conditions such as attention deficit disorder

(ADD) became a household name. What was to blame? After all, the evil "fat" had left the building.

The problem is that "fat-free" does not mean "sugar-free." It also does not mean "all you can eat." By cutting fat from our diets, we were missing out on many important nutrients called essential fatty acids. As their name implies, these fats are essential to our health, fitness, and fat loss.

Four Types of Fats

Not all fats are created equal. There are four basic types of fats: monounsaturated, polyunsaturated, saturated, and trans fatty acids.

1. *Monounsaturated (omega-9):* Omega-9 fatty acids, which are found in olives, hazelnuts, grape seed oils, and almonds, are a healthy and necessary type of fat. Omega-9 fats are useful in disease prevention due to a rich antioxidant content that protects us from free radicals, which are produced by our bodies as a by-product of energy production. (You will learn more about free radicals in Chapter 12).

2. *Polyunsaturated (omega-3):* Omega-3 fatty acids are found in fish such as wild salmon, albacore tuna, sardines, and mackerel. They are abundant in flaxseeds and flaxseed oil. You can also find omega-3s in egg yolks, provided the chicken was fed an omega-3–rich diet. This is why it is good to eat eggs together with *some* yolks; the protein and fat found in an organic egg is very good for you.

    Because our brains are primarily comprised of fat (approximately 60 percent), it comes as no surprise that eating healthy, omega-3 fats has been shown to improve intelligence and alleviate symptoms of depression. This point was illustrated in a 2002 study published in the *American Journal of Psychiatry.* Researchers discovered that 2 g of pure EPA (found in fish oils) significantly improved symptoms of depression in subjects whose antidepressants had stopped working.

3. *Polyunsaturated (omega-6):* Omega-6 fatty acids are more commonly found in the diets of North Americans than omega-3s. You can find them in common food staples such as vegetable oils, raw nuts, and grains. However, the type of omega-6 you should include in your diet is called gamma linolenic

acid or GLA. This fatty acid works like a natural anti-inflammatory and is found in avocados, walnuts, and seeds.

4. *Saturated fat and trans fatty acids:* Saturated fats, which are found primarily in red meat, pork, and full-fat dairy products, have been linked to many health ailments:

- Alzheimer's
- cancer
- diabetes
- heart disease
- high LDL (bad) cholesterol
- immune system disorders
- low HDL (good) cholesterol

With the exception of what occurs naturally in the organic chicken and occasional red meat you consume, there is no need for additional saturated fats in your diet and the above-mentioned foods should be eaten sparingly.

One of the worst forms of saturated fat is trans fats, which are produced when fats undergo a process called hydrogenation. Hydrogenation extends the shelf life of a product, but, unfortunately, it also destroys the natural, healthy components of fats, making them poisonous to the body. These modified fats act as anti-essential fatty acids and are implicated in cardiovascular disease. Trans fats, which are an insidious menace to your health, are hidden in many of the foods in your grocery store. Some foods that are likely to contain trans fats are:

- bread
- cakes
- chips
- cookies
- crackers
- frosting
- frozen waffles
- margarine
- pancakes

- pies
- shortening
- taco shells

Be sure to read labels and be on the look out for any hydrogenated or partially hydrogenated fats in the ingredients.

One word of caution about essential fats: Be sure not to heat the fats or expose them to light for prolonged periods. Doing so will damage the fats and destroy many of their health-promoting properties. When cooking dishes that require oil, be sure to use extra-virgin olive oil (below its smoking point). After cooking, drizzle some fresh olive oil or flaxseed oil on top of your food for added benefit.

The Fat-Fighter Diet's Approved Fats (Phase Two)
The following is a list of approved fat sources you can choose from:

- avocados
- borage oil
- flaxseeds and flaxseed oil
- grape seed oil
- olives and extra-virgin olive oil
- Omega 3 fish oil
- organic peanut or almond butter (avoid consuming non-organic peanut butter as it may contain aflatoxin, a harmful mold).
- primrose oil
- raw almonds
- raw cashews or walnuts
- seeds

Symptoms of Omega-3 Fat Deficiency
Underconsumption of omega-3 fatty acids is very common in our society. If you are experiencing any of the following conditions, you could be deficient in omega-3 essential fatty acids:

- difficulty in losing body fat
- dry, flaky skin
- dry hair and excessive hair loss

- high cortisol levels (stress)
- low energy
- painful joints
- sluggish metabolism

The best way to ensure you are getting all the essential fatty acids your body needs is to use a supplement. It is quite difficult to consume enough of the foods that contain essential fatty acids, and there are health concerns about overconsumption of tuna and salmon, two of the foods richest in this nutrient, because of toxins and pollutants. For this reason I recommend daily supplementation of essential oils. (Follow recommendations outlined on the bottle or by your health care practitioner. Please see Chapter 12 for a list of sources of high-quality omega 3 fish oil supplements.)

Essential Fatty Acid Key Points

The right fats are not only good for your overall health, they aid in building lean muscle tissue and in losing body fat as well. Eating a no-fat or very low-fat diet can lead to a host of health problems and grind your fat loss progress to a halt. However, to obtain the best possible results from your training and health improvement program, you *must* cut down on saturated fats, eliminate trans fats, and consume sufficient amounts of essential fatty acids.

PUTTING IT ALL TOGETHER: PROTEIN, CARBOHYDRATES, AND FATS

Eating is a hormonal event.

—Barry Sears

You now know what kinds of proteins, carbohydrates, and fats you should eat every day. Next you will find out how much of these macronutrients you should consume if you are interested in losing body fat, improving your health, or increasing your lean muscle and strength.

The Golden Rule: 40–30–30

To get the best possible results from your diet, it is important that the carbohydrate, protein, and fat ratios are optimal for the goal you wish to achieve. For the majority of the population, the 40–30–30 macronutrient breakdown of carbohydrates, proteins, and fats works best. In a study published by the American Dietetic Association, 29 overweight men and women were randomized to either a 1,500-calorie 40–30–30 (carbohydrate, protein, fat) diet or a 1,500-calorie 60–15–25 diet. All subjects did resistance training for one hour, three times weekly. While both groups lost significant amounts of weight, the 40–30–30 group's weight loss was primarily from body fat, while the 60–15–25 group did not achieve significant fat loss, leading researchers to conclude that the latter group's weight loss was due to a decrease in lean muscle tissue.

As stated earlier, when you are trying to lose fat, increase muscle and strength, or improve health, building and preserving lean muscle tissue and managing the hormone insulin should be at the top of your priority list. In order to do this effectively, you must consume enough protein and ensure adequate intake of fibrous and complex carbohydrates as well as essential fatty acids. Science has proven the benefits of eating meals with a macronutrient breakdown of 40 percent carbohydrates, 30 percent protein, and 30 percent fat. These benefits include the following:

1. Increased insulin stabilization with improved fat oxidation (burning)
2. Increased glucagon, an important hormone for fat burning and energy production
3. Increased muscle building and protein sparing without excess calories
4. Increased fat-burning (lipolytic) enzymes and decreased fat-storing (lipogenic) enzymes
5. Decreased LDL (bad) cholesterol and blood triglycerides and increased HDL (good) cholesterol
6. Increased testosterone and growth hormone levels

In addition, eating a diet with a 40–30–30 ratio has been proven to lower the likelihood of developing heart disease. In a recent Harvard medical study, women who followed a 40–30–30 macronutrient breakdown were 50 percent less likely to developing heart disease compared with women following the USDA Food Pyramid!

Doing the Math: How Much of Each?

A simple calculation can be done to find out exactly how much of each macronutrient there is in your 40–30–30 meal plan.

Note: 1 g of carbohydrate = 4 calories, 1 g of protein = 4 calories, 1 g of fat = 9 calories

Fat Loss

The following calorie ranges were taken from the www.ebodi.com wellness guidance system:

Women: 1,400–1,800 calories per day
Carbohydrates (40 percent) = 140–180 g
Protein (30 percent) = 105–135 g
Fats (30 percent) = 46–60 g

Men: 2,200–2,600 calories per day
Carbohydrates (40 percent) = 220–270 g
Protein (30 percent) = 165–203 g
Fats (30 percent) = 73–90 g

Healthy Lifestyle

Women: 1,900–2,100 calories per day
Carbohydrates (40 percent) = 190–210 g
Protein (30 percent) = 142–158 g
Fats (30 percent) = 63–70 g

Men: 2,700–3,000 calories per day
Carbohydrates (40 percent) = 270–300 g
Protein (30 percent) = 203–225 g
Fats (30 percent) = 90–100 g

Increase Lean Muscle and Strength

Women: 2,200– 2,500 calories per day
Carbohydrates (40 percent) = 220–250 g
Protein (30 percent) = 165–188 g
Fats (30 percent) = 73–83 g

Men: 3,100–4,000 calories per day
Carbohydrates (40 percent) = 320–400 g
Protein (30 percent) = 240–300 g
Fats (30 percent) = 107–133 g

To make things easy, I have included some delicious 40–30–30 recipes in Chapter 13. Once you get the hang of it, there will be no need for measuring or weighing. Eating in the right balance becomes second nature—and it feels great.

DON'T FORGET TO INDULGE!

While it is imperative to adhere to these guidelines most of the time, life is too short to deny yourself some pleasures. The result of your following this program will be an increased metabolic rate and an up-regulating of your body's fat-burning mechanisms. Because of this increase in your metabolism, the occasional treat will have little or no effect on your body fat percentage or on your health. As a matter of fact, indulging in your favorite treat will have a positive effect on your mind. I suggest you follow the 10 percent rule. If you eat healthy, hormonally balanced meals 90 percent of the time, the other 10 percent can be pretty much whatever you would like.

This rule is particularly helpful during certain times of the year or at social occasions where it could be misconstrued as rude to not enjoy certain foods such as birthday cakes. Do not sweat it! Consume this treat slowly, taking the time to savor each delicious morsel.

Please keep in mind that the best time to eat any "cheat" food is immediately following your resistance-training workout when your body is in the greatest need of quick-burning carbohydrates. The worst time to eat a "cheat" food is in the evening, before bed, or on days when your activity level has been low.

THE ACID–ALKALINE CONNECTION

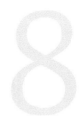

Like a swimming pool, your body has a pH level. This pH (potential for hydrogen) level must be kept in balance in order for you to become and remain lean and healthy. A pH of 6.8–7.0 is considered balanced. Anything below 6.8 is considered acidic, and anything above 7.4 is considered overly alkaline. Acid is a natural by-product of cellular metabolism. When produced in normal amounts, it poses no harm to your body and is excreted when you exhale. However, poor dietary choices and excess stress can cause your body to produce too much acid, leading to a host of health problems:

- cancer
- decreased antioxidant effectiveness
- excessive fat gain
- free radical damage
- frequent infections and colds
- headaches and muscle pain
- heart disease
- joint pain and arthritis
- low physical and mental energy
- nervousness and anxiety
- osteoporosis
- poor skin and hair
- weakened immune system

The pH of your blood, which is a different measure from your body's overall pH, is very precise and is maintained at approximately 7.3. If this pH is altered, major problems, including death, can result. For this reason, the body has multiple buffers in place to make sure the blood pH remains constant. When you are too acidic, the body neutralizes the acid with an alkaline substance, primarily sodium and calcium. The body actually takes calcium from the bones in order to neutralize blood acid. This is one of the reasons why non-organic dairy products, which are highly acid forming, are not the best choice if you are trying to reduce the risk of osteoporosis.

However, we do need to ensure that we are getting enough calcium. Recent research has shown that calcium, in addition to being important for bone health, also plays a role in fat loss. Researchers writing in the *International Journal of Obesity* found that adding an additional 300 mg of calcium to the test subjects' diet resulted in a 6 lb reduction in total body weight. In his book *The Bone-Building Solution*, researcher Sam Graci states that, "increased dietary calcium makes cells less likely to store fat and more likely to burn fat."

According to the *American Journal of Clinical Nutrition*, an alkalinizing diet will improve bone density, nitrogen balance, and growth hormone concentrations. Conversely, the low-grade acidosis resulting from an acidic diet can contribute to osteoporosis, bone loss, and a loss of muscle tissue. It is also known that cancer will thrive in an acidic environment.

Weight-related problems can also be caused by eating too many acid-forming foods. If the body cannot easily neutralize the acidic foods you eat, then it will store acid in fat cells. In addition, an acidic diet can reduce lean muscle mass (resulting in an increase in body fat) due to a decrease in growth hormone.

We must do whatever we can to tip the scales in favor of being slightly more alkaline than acidic. There are four excellent ways you can accomplish this:

1. Consume a green drink every day. These concentrated superfoods are excellent supplements. Drinking your green drink is the equivalent of consuming six full servings of alkaline-promoting vegetables in one single dose! It is so important that I recommend you start every day with this. For those people who engage in intense training, I also recommend you add a green drink supplement to your post-workout protein shake. The alkaline nature of the green drink will help to buffer the acidity inherently caused by the intense training.

2. Practise deep breathing and meditation. Feed your body and your mind more of the most vital nutrient of all—oxygen. Be mindful to breathe deeply and slowly at regular intervals throughout the day.
3. Start your day by drinking a glass of water with a squeeze of lemon. Do this on an empty stomach. Lemons are an interesting fruit. They start off being acidic, but once broken down by the body, their residue is alkaline forming. Lemon is also a natural detoxifier and will help keep your body in proper alkaline balance while assisting with digestion.
4. Eat an alkalinizing diet. To promote optimal health, the foods you eat should be approximately 75 percent alkaline forming and 25 percent acid forming. Use the following list to help you make better choices.

THE 20 MOST ALKALINE-FORMING FOODS

1. black cherries
2. black olives
3. broccoli
4. cantaloupe
5. Celtic sea salt
6. cucumber
7. garlic
8. honeydew
9. green drinks
10. kale
11. nectarine
12. onions
13. Oriental greens
14. parsley
15. raisins
16. raspberries
17. sea vegetables
18. spinach
19. watermelon
20. wheat grass and sprouts

THE 20 MOST ACID-FORMING FOODS

1. alcohol
2. artificial sweeteners
3. barley
4. cakes
5. cookies
6. cranberries
7. dried fruits
8. egg yolks
9. lobster and red meat
10. monosodium glutamate (MSG)
11. pastries
12. pistachios
13. processed and hard cheeses
14. processed soybeans
15. salted and sweetened peanut butter
16. soft drinks
17. soya sauce
18. tarts
19. trans fatty acids
20. white vinegar

ACTION
Choose foods that are both rich in nutrients and promote an alkaline blood pH.

WHAT TO DRINK

What if I told you there was a legal, abundant, and 100 percent safe substance that would improve your health, increase your strength, increase fat loss, improve your complexion, and improve your performance in any sport—without any side effects? Would you be interested? Of course! Well, there is such a substance—H_2O or, as it is more commonly called, water.

Here are some interesting facts about this miracle substance:

1. Between 60 and 70 percent of your body weight is water and you lose a large percentage of it every day through normal body processes. You body needs water for digestion, respiration, the lubrication of joints, and the transportation of nutrients. You can live quite a long while without fat, carbohydrates, or protein, but you will live only a few days without water!

2. Your body needs water for fat metabolism. When you are dehydrated (as 75 percent of the population is), your body slows the elimination of water, causing waste products to accumulate. The buildup of these waste products taxes the liver, causing it to become less efficient, thus slowing your metabolism.

3. Drinking *more* water will cause you to retain *less* water. When you deprive your body of water (much like when you deprive your body of calories), the body's reaction is to hold on to or retain water.

4. Water will fill you up, making you feel more full, which reduces your chances of overeating. Make sure you have a tall glass of water half an hour before each meal.

5. Water calms your appetite. Signals of hunger are often confused with signals of dehydration.

6. Water increases strength and endurance. Being even slightly dehydrated will decrease sports performance between 10 and 30 percent. Dehydration has also been shown to raise levels of the stress hormone cortisol.

7. The more muscle you have, the more water you will need. With the Fat-Fighter Diet, you will be adding new lean muscle to your body. Because muscle consists of more than 70 percent water, this new muscle will require extra water.

HOW MUCH WATER?

Regardless of the amount of water contained in your protein drinks and fruit juices, your body still requires a minimum of 8–10 glasses per day in addition to those other beverages. This amount should be increased if you are a person who sweats excessively or if you are training in a hot climate. Remember, thirst is a poor indicator of your level of hydration. In addition, always be sure to drink while exercising. I find it surprising to see a large number of people in the gym who do not drink while working out. They would be getting better results if they only put this simple nutrient to work for them.

ACTION

Drink fresh, clean water throughout the day. Carry a water bottle with you and keep one with you at work.

GREEN TEA: A SECRET WEAPON

I am going to let you in on a little-known secret. There is a beverage that will accelerate your metabolism while improving your health all at once. I am talking about green tea. A recent study compared the effects of green tea, caffeine, and a placebo. In this study, each subject drank either green tea (containing 150 mg of caffeine plus 375 mg of catechins), a beverage containing 150 mg caffeine, or a placebo. The results were impressive. The individuals who drank green tea with every meal burned an additional 50 calories per day than the caffeine drinkers, and 70 calories per day more than the placebo group. The reason for this is that green tea contains catechins, powerful antioxidants that, in addition to reducing your risk of cancer and heart disease, also accelerate fat loss.

While 50–70 additional calories burned may not sound like much, when you do the math, you can see the impact. Over a one-year period, this additional calorie expenditure would add up to between 18,250 to 25,550 calories burned or theoretically between 5.2 to 7.3 lbs lost—all from simply adding this health-promoting, inexpensive beverage to your daily routine.

ACTION
Drink a minimum of one cup of organic green tea each and every day.

FRUIT AND VEGETABLE JUICES

Throughout this book I have mentioned the problems associated with elevated blood sugar levels and the resulting rise in insulin. Chronic elevations in insulin can lead to diabetes and obesity. It is important that you reduce consumption of any food or beverage that elicits a dramatic rise in blood sugar levels and this includes fruit and vegetable juices. When you consume fruit and vegetable juices (without the natural skin or pulp), you are pumping pure sugar into your system. The best way to consume fruits and vegetables is in their natural state, complete with skin and pulp (this is where the fiber and much of the nutrients are contained). If you prefer to drink your fruits and vegetables, then do so with the pulp and skin intact to ensure that you receive all of the benefits without the blood sugar spike.

ACTION
Focus on eating whole fruits and vegetables (complete with skin and pulp).

WHAT ABOUT ALCOHOL?

Many of my clients have a passion for fine wine and other alcoholic beverages, and I too enjoy a glass now and then. However, if you are truly serious about losing fat and improving your health, alcohol consumption must be kept to a minimum. I cannot tell you how many times I have seen a person's fat loss goal derailed by an innocuous looking daily glass (or two) of wine. The problem is that alcohol is quite calorie dense (7 calories per gram). In addition, it is usually consumed with dinner, which consists of protein, carbohydrate, and fat calories. The liver has to work hard to metabolize the alcohol first, which suppresses the burning of the other nutrients consumed. This, combined with the added alcohol calories, is a recipe for disaster.

One argument I hear frequently is that red wine has health-promoting benefits. This is true. Red wine (not scotch, beer, or other sources of alcohol) has been shown to increase HDL (good) cholesterol while reducing LDL (bad) cholesterol. This is because red wine contains the antioxidants resveratrol and flavonoids. However, these can be obtained from other, nonalcoholic substances such as grapes, fruits, and vegetables. You can also find supplements that provide these nutrients without the added calories or toxins.

In addition, because alcohol is often mixed with sugary drinks such as cola or fruit juices, it will spike your blood sugar level. As you know, this will lead to elevated insulin, which in turn contributes to fat gain as well as a host of other health-related issues. Bingeing on alcohol will also lead to elevated cortisol levels.

In our society drinking alcohol is often part of social events. While the *occasional* glass of red wine or a cold beer now and then will have little or no effect on your body composition, the truth is alcohol is a poison and has been linked to numerous health problems, including liver disease, cancer, high blood pressure, stroke, and decreased immune function. It is also a contributor to 50 percent of all traffic fatalities. People who are serious about their health are wise to limit consumption of alcohol.

ACTION

Eliminate alcohol consumption or limit it to one or two glasses per week. Remember that alcohol has 7 calories per gram!

LET'S GO SHOPPING!

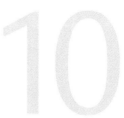

By now you have learned what foods you should eat, how much you should eat, and when you should eat. The next time you go to the grocery store, use the best and worst foods lists to quickly analyze your cart. If you see anything from the worst foods list, put them aside and know that you have taken a valuable step toward achieving your goal.

THE BEST AND WORST FOODS

The Best

In his book *The Food Connection,* nutritional researcher Sam Graci explains that the best foods are bioenergetic whole foods, which are plant-based foods grown under the direct energy pathway of the sun and infused with the energy of the soil and water. These types of foods are your best choices for optimizing health and losing body fat:

1. *Colorful vegetables:* Vegetables, including peppers, green and yellow beans, yams, broccoli, radishes, greens, beets, carrots, and many more, are great tasting and great for you. These foods are rich in nutrients and fiber and low in calories. They also contain many cancer-fighting properties.

2. *Herbs and spices:* Many herbs offer unique healing properties and health benefits, such as antioxidants and enzymes, in addition to adding flavor to many dishes.

3. *Ripe fruits:* Ripe fruits, including apples, oranges, peaches, plums, and cherries, will give your body a great antioxidant boost along with fiber, vitamins, and minerals.

4. *Berries:* These types of fruits are perhaps the healthiest of all fruits and contain powerful antioxidants, polyphenols, phytonutrients, and other anti-cancer properties. Stock up on blueberries, raspberries, strawberries, gogi berries, and blackberries.

5. *Whole grains:* Whole grains include slow-cook oatmeal, breads, flour, and pasta made from 100 percent whole grains, which are high in fiber and B-vitamins and aid in balancing blood sugar levels while providing sustained energy.

6. *Beans and legumes:* Beans and legumes, including black beans, green beans, kidney, fava, adzuki, lentils, navy, and lima beans, have been shown to be beneficial in reducing blood cholesterol and blood pressure. A report published in the *American Journal of Clinical Nutrition* states: "Beans significantly lower cholesterol levels even in high-fat diets." Beans are also rich in fiber and protein, which keep blood sugar levels balanced.

7. *Raw nuts:* Raw, unprocessed nuts such as almonds, cashews, walnuts, and macadamia nuts are high in potassium, magnesium, protein, fiber, and essential fats. Research has shown that eating a handful of raw nuts a day can lower LDL (bad) cholesterol. Roasted nuts are to be avoided. The process of roasting nuts in oil alters the composition of the fat contained within the nut changing it from a "good" fat to a "bad" fat. Be sure to avoid non-organic peanuts as they are frequently contaminated with aflatoxin, a carcinogen produced from a type of mold that often grows on peanuts.

8. *Raw seeds and sprouts:* Seeds such as sunflower, sesame, and pumpkin seeds contain essential fats and protein, while sprouts, especially alfalfa and wheat grass sprouts, contain concentrated nutrients, including protein, essential amino acids, vitamins, enzymes, and minerals.

9. *Sea vegetables:* Sea vegetables (kelp, dulse, nori, kuze, arame) are very nutrient dense, high in essential minerals and trace minerals, chlorophyll, iodine,

protein, and essential fatty acids. They have also been shown to improve thyroid function and aid in the growth of nails, hair, bones, and teeth.

10. *Greens:* Spinach, arugula, endive, romaine lettuce, mustard greens, chard, kale, dandelion greens, parsley, watercress, and green drinks are all high in chlorophyll, a potent antioxidant and phytochemical. They are also rich in vitamins and minerals, including co-enzyme Q10, which aids in strengthening the heart.

    High-quality green drinks are very nutrient dense. They contain a myriad of alkaline-forming, bioenergetic, colorful, organically grown grasses and hormone-supporting vegetables. They supply fiber, phyto-nutrients, antioxidants, and naturally occurring vitamins and minerals.

In addition to these foods, be sure to purchase protein foods. These include fish, chicken, organic eggs, shellfish, organic dairy, tempeh, tofu, extra-lean organic red meat, and protein isolates.

The Worst

You have already eliminated the following foods from your home in Phase One of the Fat Fighter Diet, and you must be diligent in not allowing them to make their way back in. Remember that the worst foods are highly refined, processed, packaged, colored, hydrogenated, and otherwise adulterated. These foods have had most of their essential nutritional elements and components removed or damaged through processing. They predispose people who eat them to fat gain, accelerated aging, negative moods, and disease.

1. *Soda pop and artificial fruit-flavored beverages:* These sugar-filled drinks are the worst choice you can make when it comes to selecting a beverage. They are full of caffeine, artificial flavors, preservatives, and sugar. They spike your blood sugar, sharply increase your acidity, add empty calories to your diet, and accelerate the aging process.

2. *Cured meats, sausages, luncheon meats, hot dogs:* These meats are a poor protein source and contain nitrites, preservatives, saturated fats, and sodium. Need I say more?

3. *Ice cream and frozen desserts:* The combination of sugar and fat makes these two of the worst foods you can consume when you are trying to lose body fat.

4. *Commercial white breads and packaged baked goods:* These products are made with refined flour and sugar, which will spike blood sugar levels. They also have little nutrient content, making them a very poor choice.

5. *Commercial breakfast cereals:* Boxed cereals usually contain partially hydrogenated oil, refined flour, and sugars. They are also loaded with artificial food dyes and preservatives.

6. *Margarine, lard, and shortening:* These are hydrogenated oils or trans fats and tend to act like saturated fats in the body. Once eaten, they destroy nutrients and make them toxic. They also raise bad cholesterol (LDL) levels and contribute to heart disease.

7. *Processed cheese products:* Highly processed and full of artificial food dyes, taste enhancers, saturated fat, and partially hydrogenated oils, these products are fake foods and have little nutrient value.

8. *Fried fast foods:* All fried fast foods are way too high in calories and contain high levels of trans fats with no nutrients whatsoever.

9. *Candy and candy bars:* These "snacks" are full of refined sugars, which will increase blood sugar levels. Chronically elevated blood sugar levels contribute to obesity, hormone imbalances, and diabetes as well as a host of other problems.

10. *Cookies and biscuits:* These "treats" contain trans fats, refined flour, and sugar and offer little or no nutrient value.

ACTION

Keep this list with you and double-check your cart the next time you go shopping.

READING LABELS

While I do advocate a 30 percent intake of healthy fats in your diet, you must always be on the lookout for hidden "bad" fats, which are often found in meat and dairy products that may be advertised as being "low fat." Do not believe everything you read! Manufacturers are quite clever at tricking you into purchasing what you believe to be a "low-fat" food, when in fact it is anything but. There is often a vast difference between label claims and what the food actually contains. Let me give you an example.

Low-fat Turkey (one slice)
30 calories
2 g fat

Looks good right? Look closer. Fat has 9 calories per gram. This "low-fat" product lists 2 g of fat: $9 \times 2 = 18$ calories from fat; $18 \div 30 = .6$ or 60 percent of calories from fat! Definitely deceiving and certainly not low fat!

You can do this with any food. Simply multiply the fat grams (per serving) by 9 and divide by the calories per serving. Make sure that you differentiate between the different types of fat and remember that not all fats are created equal. Always keep your fats to a maximum of 30 percent of your total calories.

ACTION
Prepare your shopping list before you go to the store. Read each ingredient label carefully when purchasing the foods you need.

WHY EAT ORGANIC?

You have probably noticed the word "organic" pop up more than a few times in this book. As a matter of fact, organic is one of the hottest trends going right now. But what does "organic" mean anyway?

Organic fruits and vegetables are grown without the use of pesticides, herbicides, fungicides, synthetic fertilizers, or growth-stimulating chemicals. Organic farmers generate a more nutrient-dense and fertile soil by rotating the crop each season. This encourages soil regeneration and prevents the depletion of essential nutrients. As a result, naturally strong crops grown in fertile soil will be more nutritious. Conventional farmers plant the same crops on the same soil every year, which depletes nutrient levels and results in erosion.

Organic farmers also use natural fertilizers such as manure, nutrient-dense sea kelp, and compost, all of which are produced on the farm. Pests are controlled naturally by biodegradable sprays, soaps, and other earth-friendly methods that do not alter the ecological balance. Organic farmers do not use genetically engineered plants or irradiated seeds that may be hazardous to human health.

In addition, organically farmed livestock are raised humanely and allowed to roam freely in the pasture. Livestock are given only organic feed and herd sizes are kept to a minimum to prevent overcrowding and disease. The use of growth hormones and antibiotics (routine in other forms of farming) are not permitted.

Is Organic Food More Nutrient Dense?

No one can dispute that fruits and vegetables grown without synthetic chemicals are better for our health than those coated with pesticides and other toxins. There have also been numerous studies that identify the nutritional differences between organically and conventionally grown produce.

Several studies in France and the U.K. reported that organic produce averaged higher levels of vitamins A, B, C, and E, and the minerals zinc and calcium, along with other beneficial phytonutrients. The American Chemical Society conducted studies that concluded organic oranges contained 30 percent more vitamin C than conventionally grown oranges.

The Impact on Human and Environmental Health

Synthetic fertilizers upset the soil balance and ecosystem. They add to groundwater pollution and pose a hazard to human health. It is estimated that, worldwide, several billion kilograms of pesticides are applied to crops every year. Direct and indirect exposure to pesticides (farm workers and their families, for example) have been linked to hormone disruption, cancer, and neurological disease.

The Benefits of Organic Foods

There are several benefits to eating organically grown foods:

1. Organic foods are free of toxic chemicals.
2. Organic foods are more nutritious because they are grown in nutrient-dense soil free of synthetic fertilizers.
3. Organic foods are grown without the use of irradiated seeds and genetically engineered plants.

4. Organic farming is better for the environment because it promotes soil health naturally without using synthetic fertilizers that contaminate our water.
5. Organically raised livestock are raised humanely and free of growth hormones and antibiotics.
6. Organic farmers seek to work with nature rather than to control it with chemicals.

When we consider the impact that conventional agricultural methods have on the health of the earth and on humans, and the continuing depletion of nutrients from our soil and food, it becomes obvious that organic food is our best choice.

THE TOP 10 MOST CONTAMINATED FOODS

1. apples
2. apricots
3. cantaloupes from Mexico
4. celery
5. cherries
6. grapes from Chile
7. green beans
8. peaches
9. spinach
10. strawberries

It is important that if you consume any of the above-mentioned foods, make sure they are organic because the conventional counterparts have unacceptable levels of pesticides and fungicides.

ACTION
When shopping, try to choose organic selections. Be sure to thoroughly clean all fruits and vegetables (including your organics) before eating.

DINING OUT
THE FAT-FIGHTER WAY

In our fast-paced world it is often difficult to prepare and eat meals at home 100 percent of the time. In fact, according to the National Restaurant Association, 25 percent of meals are eaten outside the home. Meals eaten away from home often suffer from what we call the "Too" syndrome: too many calories, too much fat, too much sodium, too few nutrients, and too little fiber. The following Dining out Rules will provide you with all the information you need in order to make healthier choices when eating out.

DINING OUT RULES

1. When ordering salads, ask for the dressing on the side so that you can control the fat content of the meal. Stay away from creamy dressings and instead choose olive oil, freshly squeezed lemon juice, and balsamic vinegar.

2. Skip the bread and butter or tortilla chips before your meal. These add empty calories and can raise blood sugar levels very quickly, causing an increase in fat storage.

3. Do not skip meals before eating out. Often people anticipate a large meal when dining out, so they skip breakfast or lunch. This is a very bad idea because by skipping meals, you decrease your metabolism and increase fat storage, not to mention that you will tend to eat a lot more at the restaurant where the food is higher in calories and fat.

4. Always choose baked, poached, grilled, stir-fried, or broiled foods over fried and breaded foods. They are healthier choices and tend to be lower in the bad fats.

5. Avoid drinking large amounts with meals. Liquids dilute the digestive juices in your stomach, making it more difficult to digest your meals. Stay away from soda pop and diet soda due to their empty calories and artificial sweeteners. The best beverages to choose are water and green tea (which is widely available at restaurants today).

6. If you start to feel full, do not feel that you must finish the entire meal. Almost all restaurants serve portions that are larger than they need to be. Ask the wait staff for a "doggy bag" for the next day. If whole-grain alternatives for potatoes, rice, or bread are unavailable, ask them to substitute with more vegetables.

7. When ordering entrées, ask them to hold the butter, creamy sauces and dressings, oils, cheese, and bacon, or order them on the side. These little additions can add huge amounts of unhealthy calories and fat to your meal. Above all, never combine high amounts of fat with refined carbohydrates, such as fettuccine Alfredo or nachos with cheese (however, I have included a fantastic and healthy nachos and dip recipe in Chapter 13)!

8. Watch out for these items when ordering: au gratin (with cheese), creamy, crispy, and stroganoff. Entrées with these descriptions are most likely higher in fat and lower in nutrients.

9. If you crave something sweet at the end of your meal, be strong and avoid the decadent desserts. Instead, choose a fruit dish or berry bowl.

10. Chew your food thoroughly, eat slowly, and remember to use all your senses to taste and savor your food and enjoy your dining-out experience.

11. Very important! Before you eat any meal, ask yourself this key question: Will the food I am about to eat move me *closer* to my desired body and health or *further and further* down the road toward high body fat, low energy, and poor mental acuity?

DINING OUT PORTION SIZES

You may be eating healthy food choices that are both high in fiber and lower in calories and fat. However, are you eating large portions? It is very important to eat nutritious and balanced foods in order to decrease body fat, but portion size also plays an important role. When dining out, do you know how much you should be eating?

The following is an approximate guide to portion sizes per serving that are specific to you. Adhere to these guidelines to ensure that you do not consume too many calories while dining out.

Proteins

Choose chicken, turkey, lean red meat, fish, and tofu. These foods should be the size of the palm of your hand and the thickness of a deck of playing cards or an audiotape.

Tips for fat loss:: Try to incorporate protein into your diet throughout the day. Remember that protein aids in fat burning because it has a higher thermic effect than fats or carbohydrates.

Complex Carbohydrates:

Choose vegetables, wild rice, sweet potatoes, whole grains, or beans. These foods should amount to the size of your own fist (or less) when cooked.

Tips for fat loss: Try to consume more fibrous carbohydrates, such as vegetables, and reduce intake of starchy carbohydrates, such as potatoes. Eat your starchy carbohydrates earlier in the day (and immediately following exercise) so that you can burn them off throughout the day.

Essential Fatty Acids

Choose healthy oils, including flaxseed oil, sesame oil, extra-virgin olive oil, cold-water fish oil, avocado, nuts, and seeds. Generally consume 1 tbsp of oil per meal or one *small* palm-sized portion of nuts and seeds.

Tips for fat loss:: Essential fats increase thermogenesis or weight loss through heat generation. EFAs will also help to balance blood sugar levels and are satiating, helping you to feel full.

ACTION

Remember these rules and always watch portion sizes whenever (and wherever) you eat away from home.

SUPPLEMENTATION

Before we begin discussing supplements, I would like to say that, first and foremost, food is the most important source for nutrients and the backbone of your nutrition plan. Supplements are just that—supplements. They are meant to be an addition to your healthy, Fat-Fighter Diet, not in place of it.

That said, supplements can help balance your body systems and assist you in achieving your health and fitness goals. The nutrient quality of our foods is continually declining due to agricultural practices, soil erosion, preservatives, genetically modified foods, and pollutants. As such, it can be beneficial to supplement our diets in order to obtain essential vitamins and minerals that may be lacking from our food.

Vitamins and minerals are nutrients that the body requires in small amounts in order to perform vital functions. A well-balanced diet rich in organic vegetables, fruits, and lean proteins could possibly give your body all the vitamins and minerals it needs, provided that the soil the fruits and vegetables were grown in and the plants the animals ate were rich in minerals themselves. However, with increased demand put on your body through exercise, work, and stress, there is a greater need for nutrients. Because it is very difficult to eat "perfectly" all of the time, it makes sense to supplement your daily diet with a quality vitamin and mineral supplement. Dr. Jonathan Prousky, ND, chief naturopathic medical officer and associate professor of clinical nutrition at the Canadian College of Naturopathic Medicine, agrees that, "all adults should take a good multivitamin and multimineral because we can't get all the nutrients we need from our diet." Vitamin deficiency is actually quite common, especially in the elderly.

BUILDING THE CASE: WHY YOU SHOULD USE SUPPLEMENTS

The following are some compelling examples of the poor nutritive quality of common foods that will help drive home the importance of using high-quality dietary supplements.

Fruits and vegetables in Canadian grocery stores contain fewer nutrients today than they used to:

Research by CTV, published in *The Globe and Mail*, shows that broccoli contains 62 percent less calcium; potatoes have lost almost all their vitamin A; and apples have lost nearly half their iron. In all, among the majority of fruits and vegetables tested, there was a 68 percent loss of vitamin A, a 76 percent loss of iron, and an 80 percent loss of calcium. (Source: CTV.ca July 6, 2002)

Similar findings regarding U.S.-grown fruits and vegetables were published by Life Extension(www.lef.org) in 2001:

Since 1975 in the U.S., there has been a 50 percent reduction in the calcium found in broccoli; cauliflower is down 40 percent in vitamin C; watercress is down 88 percent in iron; and vitamin A in apples dropped from 90 mg to 53 mg. In a 1996 study conducted by the U.S Department of Agriculture (U.S.D.A), researcher Linda Scott-Kantor revealed that iceberg lettuce, processed tomato, onion, and potato account for 50 percent of vegetable intake among adults.

In the same year Larry Craig, writing in the *Journal of the American Dietetic Association,* discovered that an average adult eats only 1.5 servings of vegetables per day and less than one serving of fruit per day. Only one out of 11 adults eats three servings of vegetables and two servings of fruit daily, which is still very low. One out of nine adults eats no fruit and vegetables on a given day.

In the July 5, 2002 edition of *The Globe and Mail*, Dr. Walter Willet, chairman of the Department of Nutrition at Harvard, declared "a daily multivitamin is a good, cheap insurance policy" and states that the Canada Food Guide should include a recommendation that supplements be included as part of a healthy diet as they are important to ensure adequate levels of folic acid and vitamins B6, B12, D, and E.

The poor nutrient quality of the foods we consume can lead to a variety of health conditions. Supplementation can help address this problem. In light of these findings, I recommend that all of my clients take a potent multivitamin/ multimineral as well as a green drink each and every day.

ANTIOXIDANTS AND FREE RADICALS: THE BATTLE RAGES ON

Free radicals may sound like the name of a new rock group, but in fact they are much more sinister. Homeopathic doctor Bryce Wylde offers a compelling explanation of what exactly free radicals are, why you should be concerned about them, and what you can do to combat free radical damage.

According to Dr. Wylde, "free radicals are also known as oxidants, which are the byproducts of oxygen that is burnt every time we breathe in a lung full of air. A normal oxygen molecule has four pairs of electrons. Through our daily metabolism and other mechanisms, a molecule sometimes loses one of its electrons and thereby becomes incomplete and more reactive. This unstable oxygen molecule is called a free radical. A free radical aggressively attacks and steals electrons from other oxygen atoms in order to balance itself. This causes other hijacked molecules to lose stability, subsequently leading to a chain reaction of free radicals. To counter free radicals (or oxidants), our body needs antioxidants, which supply the needed electrons to stop the chain reaction process."

Dr. Wylde likens the damage caused by free radicals in our bodies to that of the oxidation that causes metal to rust. To prevent rusting, we apply rust paint, and antioxidants do something similar for our bodies.

Left unchecked, free radical damage can lead to impaired fat loss, accelerated aging, and disease. Because free radical production takes place in the muscles' mitochondrion (your fat-burning epicenter), it is important to protect your mitochondrion from their attack. By taking a good-quality daily multivitamin/multimineral, you will help to ensure your body is receiving the necessary antioxidants (mainly vitamins C, E, A, and coenzyme Q10) and the appropriate antioxidant levels. This is especially important for people who exercise, who are under emotional stress, who are exposed to pollution, and for those who drink, smoke, or eat fried foods. I think this covers just about everyone!

SUPPLEMENT RECOMMENDATIONS

I have included the following supplement recommendations for you to follow. Everybody should follow the Healthy Lifestyle supplement plan. If you have additional goals such as fat loss or increasing lean muscle and strength, then I would encourage you to include those supplements in addition to the Healthy Lifestyle supplements outlined below. *Please remember to always consult with your physician before beginning any supplement program. For specific product recommendations, please turn to the product resources section at the end of the book.*

Healthy Lifestyle

Omega-3 Fatty Acids (Fish Oil)

Omega-3 fatty acids are very beneficial to your overall health and wellness. In fact, fish oil tops my list when it comes to supplements we can all benefit from using. These benefits include:

1. An increase in thermogenesis (loss of energy as heat)
2. A decrease in body fat mass and fat cell volume
3. The turning on of genes associated with burning of abdominal fat (lipolytic genes)
4. The turning off of genes associated with storage of body fat (lipogenic genes)
5. A reduction in inflammation, which can result from intense physical training
6. A reduction in stress hormone production (cortisol)
7. Regulation of brain areas that are responsible for a feeling of fullness
8. A reduction in the risk of developing diabetes, heart disease, and stroke
9. Support for health conditions such as diabetes, emotional disorders, gastrointestinal disorders, pregnancy, inflammatory conditions, menstrual discomfort, and skin conditions such as psoriasis and eczema

Look for a fish oil supplement with a high percentage of EPA (eicosapentaenoic acid). With fish oils (as with everything else), you get what you pay for. Be sure to check the percentage of EPA and DHA (docosahexaenoic acid) on the label and buy from a reputable manufacturer.

Green Drink

Green drinks are right up there with fish oils when it comes to foundational supplements. These amazing beverages help to increase energy levels, improve memory, improve overall brain function, improve digestion, and balance pH levels. Green drinks boost your immune system and are packed full of phytonutrients. Green drinks also contain phosphatidyl serine (PS), a phospholipid that appears to have cortisol-suppressing properties, which is great for fat loss.

If you have never used a green drink before, start by using it only once per day. Once your system has become accustomed to taking a green drink (usually after five to seven days), increase to using one serving in the morning and another immediately following an intense workout. The post-workout green drink will help to buffer the acidity caused by the intense training and shift your body back toward a more alkaline state.

Multivitamin and Mineral Complex

A multivitamin and mineral complex is needed for proper immune function, growth and development, antioxidant status, and metabolism. It is also known that nutrient deficiencies may contribute to obesity. This daily supplement aids in the proper functioning of the immune system, supports cardiovascular and bone health, is important for growth and development, adds to antioxidant status, and supports adequate levels of micronutrients to protect against chronic disease.

Make sure that you are getting enough vitamin C. Studies have shown a reduction in cortisol levels in intense exercisers who take 1,000 mg of vitamin C per day. Vitamin C may also reduce pain and speed recovery following intense exercise. In addition, vitamin C may also help prevent exercise-related muscle injuries by neutralizing free radicals produced during strenuous exercise.

Fat Loss

If your goal is fat loss, include the following supplements in addition to your Healthy Lifestyle supplement plan.

Conjugated Linoleic Acid (CLA)

CLA helps decrease both the size and volume of fat cells, particularly around the abdomen. It may also assist in maintaining muscle mass while decreasing overall body fat. CLA helps to balance both blood sugar and the hormone insulin.

Green Tea (Standardized Epigallocatechin gallate or EGCG)

Green tea can increase fat breakdown and support weight loss. Research shows that green tea safely enhances thermogenesis, increasing 24-hour energy expenditure and fat burning. Green tea also contains potent antioxidants and is beneficial for heart health.

Hydroxycitric acid (HCA)

HCA curbs appetite, inhibits the conversion of carbohydrates into fat, reduces fat production and storage, and improves the rate of fat burning in cells.

R-Alpha Lipoic Acid

R-alpha lipoic acid is a powerful antioxidant and quenches free radicals. Research has shown that free radicals cause extensive muscle damage and play a major role in accelerated aging, disease, and death. In addition to fighting free radicals,

R-alpha lipoic acid improves insulin sensitivity, enabling the body to utilize insulin more efficiently, which leads to stable blood sugar levels and improved fat loss.

Fiber

Several trials have shown that supplementation with fiber from various sources accelerates weight loss. Fiber slows down the absorption of fat through the small intestines, which leads to a sense of fullness and can help curb appetite.

Increase Lean Muscle and Strength

If your current goal is to increase lean muscle and strength, include the following supplements in addition to your Healthy Lifestyle supplement plan.

Whey Protein Isolate

Whey protein isolate is best taken after weight training to enhance the rate of repair and rebuilding of muscle tissue. Whey protein isolate or a blend of casein (milk) and whey protein (which is slower to digest than pure whey) can also be taken as a snack between meals to balance blood sugar levels and boost your metabolism. Whey protein has benefits beyond muscle building—it also improves your health. Quality whey proteins will also boost your body's production of glutathione, a powerful antioxidant. This remarkable protein has also been shown to increase immune system function due to its high levels of the amino acid L-cysteine.

Creatine Monohydrate

Creatine has been shown to increase muscle mass, especially when accompanied by exercise. Creatine can improve performance and delay muscle fatigue during high-intensity, short-duration exercise. It is also beneficial to your health. Researchers found that by supplementing with creatine (approximately 5g per day), subjects incurred a reduction in blood levels of homocysteine, an amino acid that has been linked to heart disease.

ACTION
Purchase the supplements that correspond to your goal. Follow the directions as recommended by the manufacturer or those of your health care practitioner.

TRANSFORM WORDS INTO ACTION!

To Do List:

- Eat regulary and never drastically cut calories.
- Focus on percent body fat, not BMI or scale weight alone.
- Cleanse your kitchen and body.
- Calculate how much food is right for *you.*
- Take the steps necessary to become more alkaline and less acidic.
- Always eat breakfast and never skip meals!
- Eat three meals and two snacks every day.
- Drink one or more cups of green tea daily.
- Do not eat after eight in the evening.
- Drink plenty of fresh water.
- Choose supplements according to your goal.
- Read this list daily as a reminder of what you *must* do to achieve your goal!

There you have it. You are now well versed on the subject of nutrition as it relates to optimizing your health, metabolism, and fat loss. You have learned why your last diet (like most diets) failed, and the critical importance of focusing on *fat* loss, not just *weight* loss. By now you should have a clearly defined outcome goal that you wish to achieve as well as behavior goals to support you in your quest. You now know exactly what, when, how often, and how much you should eat according to your goal, and you understand the important role that cleansing plays in the process. You know the importance of green tea and the problem with sugar-laden foods and beverages. You also understand that all calories are not created equally, and why simply reducing your calories (as advocated in most mainstream diets) is a recipe for failure.

You also have an impressive understanding of proteins, carbohydrates, and fats. You can now go to the supermarket and decipher those misleading label claims while choosing the best foods for you and your family. Lastly, you have discovered how to dine out without "blowing" your diet, and what supplements will speed up your results and improve your health. If you turn to the next chapter, you will even have a new roster of fabulous recipes, all designed in the 40–30–30 ratio and tailored to your specific daily calorie requirements!

However, class is not over yet. We have one more thing to talk about—exercise.

In the next chapters you are going to learn why exercise is an important part of the holistic lifestyle. I will then give you a fitness test to assess your present fitness level and provide you with a detailed resistance training, flexibility, and cardio program to help you succeed in achieving your goal.

THE PERFECT PLATE

I have included the following sample one-week fat loss meal plan for you to enjoy. Each one of these recipes is balanced to include 40 percent of calories from healthy carbohydrates, 30 percent from lean protein, and 30 percent from healthy fats. This hormone-friendly ratio will help propel you to your fat loss goal! To begin, please refer to Chapter 7 to determine your caloric allotment. Once you have calculated your body's caloric requirements for the day, simply follow the recipe quantities under your calorie group (1,200–2,800). You can find hundreds more like this, all perfectly portioned for your body and your goals at www.ebodi.com.

Note: Each of the following recipes makes one serving for each calorie group.

BREAKFAST

Active Life Oatmeal

Ingredients	1200	1400	1600	1800	2000	2200	2400	2600	2800
Banana, sliced	¼	¼	¼	⅓	⅓	½	½	½	½
Whey protein powder (tbsp)	3½	4	5	5	6	6½	7	7½	8
Cinnamon (tsp)	1	1	1	1½	2	2	2	2	2
Slow-cook oats (cup)	½	½	½	⅔	⅔	¾	¾	1	1
Walnuts, chopped (cup)	⅛	⅛	⅛	⅛	⅛	¼	¼	¼	¼

Directions: In a pot add the banana, whey protein powder, and cinnamon to the oatmeal. Cook over medium heat for five minutes, stirring often. Top with walnuts and enjoy!

Apple and Oatmeal Pancakes

Ingredients	1200	1400	1600	1800	2000	2200	2400	2600	2800
Apples with skin, diced (cup)	⅓	⅓	½	½	½	⅔	⅔	¾	¾
Instant oats (cup)	½	½	⅔	¾	¾	1	1	1	1
Whey protein powder (tbsp)	1½	2	2	2	2½	3	3	3	4
Cinnamon (tsp)	½	½	1	1	1	1	1	1	1
Stevia (tsp)	½	½	1	1	1	1	1	1	1

Directions: Dice apples into small pieces. Combine all ingredients and mix together in a bowl. Warm a non-stick frying pan to medium heat. Add mixture and cook until brown on each side. Enjoy!

Berry Oat Bran

Ingredients	1200	1400	1600	1800	2000	2200	2400	2600	2800
Oat bran (cup)	¾	1	1	1⅛	1¼	1⅓	1½	1⅔	1¾
Rice Dream beverage (fl oz)	¼	¼	¼	⅓	⅓	½	½	½	½
Blueberries (cup)	⅛	⅛	⅛	⅛	¼	¼	¼	¼	⅓
Almonds, whole (cup)	⅛	⅛	¼	¼	¼	¼	⅓	⅓	⅓
Whey protein powder (tbsp)	3½	4	5	5	6	6½	7	7½	8
Raisins (cup)	⅛	⅛	⅛	⅛	⅛	⅛	⅛	⅛	⅛

Directions: Place oat bran in a glass or ceramic bowl and add double the amount of boiling water. Cover with a lid and let sit for 15 minutes or until desired consistency is achieved. Remove lid and add rice milk, followed by all other ingredients. Enjoy!

Egg White Omelet

Ingredients	1200	1400	1600	1800	2000	2200	2400	2600	2800
Egg whites, large	4	5	5	6	7	7	8	9	9
Broccoli, chopped (cup)	2	2½	3	3	3	4	4	4	5
Extra-virgin olive oil (tbsp)	⅔	¾	1	1	1⅛	1¼	1⅓	1½	1½
Red peppers, chopped (cup)	1	1⅛	1⅓	1½	1⅔	1¾	2	2⅛	2⅓
Spinach, chopped (cup)	1¼	1½	1⅔	1¾	2	2¼	2½	2⅔	2¾
Cherry tomatoes, halved (cup)	1¼	1½	1⅔	1¾	2	2¼	2½	2⅔	2¾

Directions: In a bowl, combine egg whites. Lightly coat a nonstick pan with olive oil. Add vegetables and cook on medium heat until tender. Pour egg mixture on top. Reduce heat and cook each side of the omelet for five minutes. Enjoy!

Scrambled Eggs

Ingredients	1200	1400	1600	1800	2000	2200	2400	2600	2800
Extra-virgin olive oil (tbsp)	¼	¼	⅓	⅓	½	½	½	½	½
Green onions, chopped (cup)	1	1½	1½	1½	2	2	2	2	2
Red peppers, sliced (cup)	½	½	⅔	¾	¾	1	1	1⅛	1⅛
Mushrooms, medium, sliced	4	5	5	6	7	7	8	9	10
Egg white, large	3	3	4	4	5	5	6	6	7
Cherry tomatoes, halved (cup)	1¼	1½	1⅔	1¾	2	2¼	2½	2⅔	2¾
Whole egg, small	1	1	1	2	3	4	4	5	5
Sea salt (tsp)	¼	¼	⅓	⅓	½	½	½	½	½
Soy sauce (tbsp)	1	1⅛	1⅓	1½	1⅔	1¾	2	2⅛	2⅓
Curry powder (tsp)	¼	¼	⅓	⅓	½	½	½	½	½
Cayenne pepper (tsp)	⅛	⅛	⅛	⅛	¼	¼	¼	¼	⅓
Turmeric (tsp)	⅛	⅛	⅛	⅛	¼	¼	¼	¼	⅓
Whole-grain bread (slices)	1½	2	2	2½	2½	3	3	3	3½
Tomatoes, sliced	1	1	1	1	1	1	1	2	2

Directions: Preheat a frying pan with olive oil. Sauté onion, red pepper, and mushrooms for about two minutes. Add the eggs, sea salt, soy sauce, curry powder, cayenne pepper, and turmeric and scramble the mixture. Mix thoroughly until the color is consistent. Sauté for three to six minutes more until the flavors mingle and the mixture is hot throughout. Serve immediately with toasted rye bread and tomato slices. Enjoy!

Granola Yogurt

Ingredients	1200	1400	1600	1800	2000	2200	2400	2600	2800
Ready-to-eat granola (cup)	⅛	⅛	⅛	⅛	¼	¼	¼	¼	¼
Flaxseed oil (tbsp)	½	½	½	⅔	⅔	¾	¾	1	1
Plain organic low-fat yogurt (cup)	1⅓	1½	1¾	2	2¼	2½	2⅔	3	3¼

Directions: Add granola and flaxseed oil to yogurt and enjoy.

Muesli

Ingredients	1200	1400	1600	1800	2000	2200	2400	2600	2800
Muesli (cup)	¼	¼	⅓	⅓	½	½	½	½	½
Whey protein powder (tbsp)	3	3½	4	4½	5	5½	6	6½	7
Ground flaxseeds (tbsp)	2	2½	3	3	3½	4	4	4½	5
Plain organic low-fat yogurt (cup)	⅓	⅓	½	½	½	⅔	⅔	¾	¾

Directions: Mix all ingredients together. Enjoy!

MORNING SNACK

Apple and Nuts

Ingredients	1200	1400	1600	1800	2000	2200	2400	2600	2800
Apple with skin (cup)	½	½	1	1	1	1	1	1	1
Soy nuts (cup)	¼	¼	¼	⅓	⅓	½	½	½	½

Directions: Enjoy soy nuts together with your fruit.

Super Protein Shake

Ingredients	1200	1400	1600	1800	2000	2200	2400	2600	2800
Plain organic low-fat yogurt (cup)	⅓	⅓	½	½	½	½	⅔	⅔	¾
Blueberries (cup)	¼	¼	⅓	⅓	½	½	½	½	½
Fresh or canned peaches, halves or slices (cup)	¼	¼	¼	⅓	⅓	½	½	½	½
Ice cubes	2	2	2	2	3	3	3	3	3
Spring water (cup)	1	1⅛	1⅓	1½	1⅔	1¾	2	2⅛	2⅓
Whey protein powder (tbsp)	1½	2	2	2	2½	3	3	3	3½
Flaxseed oil (tbsp)	½	½	½	½	1	1	1	1	1

Directions: In a blender, combine yogurt, blueberries, peaches, ice, and water. Blend well. Add whey protein powder and flaxseed oil and blend on low for an additional 10 seconds. Enjoy!

Fiber Boost

Ingredients	1200	1400	1600	1800	2000	2200	2400	2600	2800
Flaxseed oil (tbsp)	½	½	½	1	1	1	1	1	1
Whey protein powder (tbsp)	2½	3	3	4	4	4½	5	5½	6
Spring water (cup)	1	1⅛	1⅓	1½	1⅔	1¾	2	2⅛	2⅓
Prune(s)	1	1	1	1½	2	2	2	2	2
Apple with skin (cup)	½	½	1	1	1	1	1	1	1

Directions: In a shaker cup, mix the flaxseed oil and whey protein powder with water. Shake vigorously. Enjoy with the prune(s) and apple.

Fruit and Cheese

Ingredients	1200	1400	1600	1800	2000	2200	2400	2600	2800
Grapes (cup)	¾	1	1	1⅛	1¼	1⅓	1½	1⅔	1¾
Soy cheddar cheese (slices)	3	3	4	4	4½	5	5½	6	6½

Directions: Enjoy cheese with fruit.

Fruit and Seed Snack

Ingredients	1200	1400	1600	1800	2000	2200	2400	2600	2800
Apple with skin, diced (cup)	½	½	½	½	½	½	½	½	½
Plain organic low-fat yogurt (cup)	⅔	¾	¾	1	1	1	1¼	1½	1½
Raw pumpkin seeds (cup)	⅛	⅛	⅛	⅛	⅛	⅛	⅛	⅛	⅛
Sesame seeds (tbsp)	½	½	½	½	½	½	½	½	½

Directions: Add apple to yogurt and stir. Add all other ingredients and mix. Enjoy!

Granola and Cottage Cheese

Ingredients	1200	1400	1600	1800	2000	2200	2400	2600	2800
Non-fat cottage cheese (cup)	⅓	½	½	½	⅔	¾	¾	¾	1
Granola bar	1	1	1	1	1½	1½	2	2	2

Directions: Enjoy together.

LUNCH

Chicken Wrap

Ingredients	1200	1400	1600	1800	2000	2200	2400	2600	2800
Apple with skin (cup)	½	½	½	1	1	1	1	1	1
Chicken breast, chopped or diced (cup/ounces)	½/ 2.4	½/ 2.4	½/ 2.4	⅔/ 3.2	⅔/ 3.2	¾/ 3.6	¾/ 3.6	1/ 4.8	1/ 4.8
Raw onions, chopped (tbsp)	½	½	⅔	¾	¾	1	1	1⅛	1⅛
Tomatoes, diced (cup)	½	½	½	½	¾	1	1	1	1
Organic soy mayonnaise (tbsp)	½	½	½	½	1	1	1	1	1
Whole-wheat tortilla	1	1	1	1	1	1	2	2	2
Mixed greens (cup)	½	½	⅔	¾	¾	1	1	1½	1½
Soy cheese, grated (ounces)	½	½	⅔	¾	¾	1	1	1	1

Directions: For optimal digestion, eat the apple 20–30 minutes before the rest of the meal. Bake chicken in oven at 350°F for 30 minutes or until done. Chop chicken, onion, and tomato into bite-size pieces. Spread mayonnaise over tortilla. Cover with chicken, mixed greens, soy cheese, onion, and tomato. Wrap like a fajita and enjoy!

Chicken Sandwich

Ingredients	1200	1400	1600	1800	2000	2200	2400	2600	2800
Salsa (tbsp)	2	2	3	3	3	3	4	4	4
Broccoli, chopped (cup)	¼	¼	⅓	⅓	½	½	½	½	½
Red pepper, sliced (cup)	¼	¼	⅓	⅓	½	½	½	½	½
Cooked chicken breast, diced (cup/ounces)	½/ 2.4	½/ 2.4	½/ 2.4	⅔/ 3.2	⅔/ 3.2	¾/ 3.6	¾/ 3.6	1/ 4.8	1/ 4.8
Celery, diced (cup)	¼	¼	⅓	⅓	½	½	½	½	½
Onions, diced	¼	¼	⅓	⅓	½	½	½	½	½
Soy mayonnaise (tbsp)	1	1	1	1	1	1	1	1	1½
Pumpernickel bread (slices)	2	2	2	2	2	2	3	3	3
Tomatoes, sliced	1	1	1	1	1	2	2	2	2

Directions: Use salsa as a dip for the broccoli and red pepper. Cut the chicken into small chunks. Next, dice celery and onions, and mix with mayonnaise. Add the chicken and spread the mixture on pumpernickel bread and cover with tomato slices. Enjoy!

Mediterranean Chicken Salad

Ingredients	1200	1400	1600	1800	2000	2200	2400	2600	2800
Cooked chicken breast (grams/oz.)	42/ 1.5	42/ 1.5	63/ 2.2	75/ 2.6	84/ 3	84/ 3	94.5/ 3.3	105/ 3.7	105/ 3.7
Cucumber, diced (cup)	½	½	⅔	¾	¾	1	1	1⅛	1⅛
Lettuce, shredded (cup)	1¼	1½	1⅔	2	2⅛	2¼	2½	2¾	3
Tomato wedges	6	7	8	9	10	11	12	13	14
Olives (small)	2	2	3	3	3	3	4	4	5
Extra-virgin olive oil (tbsp)	⅓	⅓	½	½	½	⅔	⅔	¾	¾
Feta cheese, crumbled (grams/oz.)	12/ 0.4	12/ 0.4	19/ 0.7	19/ 0.7	19/ 0.7	25/ 0.9	25/ 0.9	28/ 1	28/ 1
Rye bread (slices)	2	2	2	2	3	3	3	4	4

Directions: On a large plate, arrange chicken, cucumber, lettuce, tomatoes, and olives. Top with olive oil and feta cheese. Enjoy with rye bread.

Egg Salad

Ingredients	1200	1400	1600	1800	2000	2200	2400	2600	2800
Egg white (cup)	⅓	½	½	½	⅔	¾	¾	¾	1
Whole egg (large)	1	1	1	1	2	2	2	2	2
Organic soy mayonnaise (tbsp)	⅓	½	½	½	⅔	¾	¾	¾	1
Paprika (tsp)	⅛	⅛	⅛	⅛	¼	¼	¼	¼	⅓
Cayenne pepper (tsp)	⅛	⅛	⅛	⅛	¼	¼	¼	¼	⅓
Herbal seasoning (tsp)	¼	¼	⅓	⅓	½	½	½	½	½
Kelp powder (tbsp)	⅛	⅛	⅛	⅛	¼	¼	¼	¼	⅓
Red peppers, finely chopped (cup)	¼	¼	¼	⅓	⅓	½	½	½	½
Celery, finely chopped (stalk)	⅔	¾	1	1	1	1	1½	1½	1½
Spelt bread (slices)	2	2	3	3	3	4	4	4	5

Directions: Boil the eggs, putting aside one whole egg. Remove and discard the yolks of the others, reserving the whites. Mix with the mayonnaise and spices until they are finely mashed. Then add the red pepper and celery and mix. Spread on bread. Enjoy!

Salmon Sandwich

Ingredients	1200	1400	1600	1800	2000	2200	2400	2600	2800
Salmon (can)	⅛	¼	¼	¼	⅓	⅓	⅓	½	½
Organic soy mayonnaise (tbsp)	¼	¼	¼	⅓	⅓	⅓	½	½	½
Rye bread (slices)	2	2	3	3	3	4	4	4	5

Directions: Mix salmon with mayonnaise and spread on bread. Enjoy!

Turkey Sandwich

Ingredients	1200	1400	1600	1800	2000	2200	2400	2600	2800
Kiwi	1½	1½	2	2	2	2½	3	3	3
Celery, chopped (cup)	¼	¼	¼	¼	¼	¼	¼	¼	¼
Cucumber, chopped	¼	¼	¼	¼	¼	¼	¼	¼	¼
Soy mayonnaise (tbsp)	1	1	1	1	1	1	1	1	1½
Cooked turkey breast meat (grams/oz.)	63/ 2.2	84/ 3	84/ 3	105/ 3.7	105/ 3.7	126/ 4.4	126/ 4.4	147/ 5.2	147/ 5.2
Rye bread (slice)	2	2	3	3	3	4	4	4	5

Directions: For optimal digestion, eat the kiwi alone 20–30 minutes before other food. Combine celery, cucumber, and mayonnaise. Spread on the bread and top with turkey. Enjoy!

DINNER

Grilled Salmon

Ingredients	1200	1400	1600	1800	2000	2200	2400	2600	2800
Long-grain brown rice (cup)	¼	¼	¼	⅓	⅓	⅓	½	½	½
Wild salmon (oz.)	3	3½	4	4½	5	5½	6	6½	7
Lemon juice (fl oz)	¼	¼	¼	⅓	⅓	½	½	½	½
Extra-virgin olive oil (tbsp)	¼	¼	⅓	⅓	½	½	½	½	½
Asparagus	3	3	4	4½	5	5½	6	6½	7
Garlic cloves, chopped	1	1	1	1½	2	2	2	2	2
Herbal seasoning (tsp)	¼	¼	⅓	⅓	½	½	½	½	½

Directions: Cook rice according to the package instructions. Cut the salmon crosswise into 1-inch slices, then place them in the lemon juice, turning a few times. Top with some of the chopped garlic. Set aside. In a large skillet, heat the olive oil. Add asparagus and the rest of the garlic and stir until they are coated with oil. Cover and cook for five minutes until almost tender and set aside in a covered serving dish. Grill salmon and serve with the rice and asparagus. Top with herbal seasoning. Enjoy!

Chicken à la Skew

Ingredients	1200	1400	1600	1800	2000	2200	2400	2600	2800
Long-grain brown rice (cup)	⅛	¼	¼	¼	⅓	⅓	⅓	⅓	½
Chicken breast (skin and bone removed)	½	½	½	½	⅔	⅔	¾	¾	¾
Celery, chopped (cup)	¼	⅛	⅛	⅛	¼	¼	¼	¼	⅓
Mushrooms, whole	3	3	3	3	3	3	3	3	3
Onions, chopped (cup)	⅛	⅛	⅛	⅛	¼	¼	¼	¼	⅓
Red peppers, chopped (cup)	⅛	⅛	⅛	⅛	¼	¼	¼	¼	⅓
Zucchini, chopped (cup)	⅛	⅛	⅛	⅛	¼	¼	¼	¼	⅓
Extra-virgin olive oil (tbsp)	½	1	1	1	1	1	1	1	1

Directions: Cook rice as per package instructions. Cut chicken and vegetables into bite-sized chunks. Thread on a skewer. Broil for 20 minutes, turning several times. With the leftover oil, baste chicken a couple of times. Enjoy!

Stuffed Turkey Breast

Ingredients	1200	1400	1600	1800	2000	2200	2400	2600	2800
Whole grain bread crumbs (cup)	⅛	⅛	¼	¼	¼	¼	⅓	⅓	⅓
Cranberry sauce (cup)	⅛	⅛	⅛	⅛	⅛	⅛	¼	¼	¼
Extra-virgin olive oil (tbsp)	⅛	⅛	¼	¼	¼	¼	⅓	⅓	⅓
Orange juice (cup)	⅛	⅛	⅛	⅛	⅛	⅛	¼	¼	¼
Rosemary (tsp)	½	½	⅔	¾	¾	1	1	1⅛	1⅛
Sea salt (tsp)	⅛	⅛	⅛	⅛	¼	¼	¼	¼	¼
Pepper (tsp)	⅛	⅛	⅛	⅛	¼	¼	¼	¼	¼
Turkey breast (grams/oz.)	42/ 1.5	63/ 2.2	63/ 2.2	63/ 2.2	84/ 3	84/ 3	105/ 3.7	105/ 3.7	105/ 3.7
Whole egg (large)	1	1	1	2	2	2	2	2	2

Directions: Preheat oven to 300°F. Mix half of the bread crumbs with the orange juice, rosemary, sea salt, and pepper. Slice a pocket into the side of each turkey breast and stuff with bread mixture. Whisk the egg(s) in a large bowl. Sprinkle the other half of the bread crumbs onto a plate. Dip stuffed turkey breasts into the egg mixture (holding carefully so that the stuffing does not fall out) and then coat with the bread crumbs and sprinkle with olive oil. Place the stuffed and breaded turkey breasts onto a greased baking dish and cover. Bake at 300 F for 45 minutes and then remove the cover and bake for an additional 12–20 minutes until golden brown. Serve with cranberry sauce. Enjoy!

Chinese Stir-Fry

Ingredients	1200	1400	1600	1800	2000	2200	2400	2600	2800
Long-grain brown rice (cup)	⅛	⅛	⅛	⅛	⅛	⅛	¼	¼	¼
Soy sauce (tbsp)	½	½	⅔	⅔	¾	¾	1	1	1⅛
Sesame oil (tsp)	½	½	½	⅔	⅔	¾	¾	1	1
Onions or scallions, chopped (cup)	⅛	⅛	⅛	⅛	¼	¼	¼	¼	¼
Ginger, grated (tsp)	1	1	1½	2	2	2	2	2	2
Tofu, firm, grated (slices)	3½	4	4½	5	6	6	7	7	8
Carrots, grated (cup)	⅛	⅛	⅛	⅛	¼	¼	¼	¼	¼
Broccoli, chopped (cup)	⅛	⅛	⅛	⅛	¼	¼	¼	¼	¼
Water chestnuts, sliced (cup)	⅛	⅛	⅛	⅛	¼	¼	¼	¼	¼
Bean sprouts (cup)	⅛	⅛	⅛	⅛	¼	¼	¼	¼	¼
Garlic, chopped (clove)	½	½	⅔	⅔	¾	¾	1	1	1⅛

Directions: Cook rice as per instructions on package. Heat the sesame oil in a large frying pan or wok until the oil is quite warm but not hot enough to smoke or sputter. Add the chopped onions or scallions, and sauté till they are soft (about five minutes). Add the grated ginger, tofu, and carrots. Sauté until the tofu is lightly browned (about 10 minutes). Push the tofu and carrots to the side of the pan. Add the broccoli and water chestnuts, and garlic, and sauté for two minutes. Then add the bean sprouts and sauté another two minutes. Place on a bed of rice, add soy sauce to taste. Enjoy!

Chicken and Veggies

Ingredients	1200	1400	1600	1800	2000	2200	2400	2600	2800
Asparagus	4	4⅔	5⅓	6	6⅔	7⅓	8	8⅔	9⅓
Brussels sprouts	3	3½	4	4½	5	5½	6	6½	7
Walnut oil (tsp)	½	½	½	⅔	⅔	¾	¾	1	1
Pumpkin seeds (cup)	⅛	⅛	⅛	⅛	⅛	⅛	¼	¼	¼
Sweet potato	1	1	1	1	1½	1½	1¾	1¾	2
Chicken breast, boneless and skinless	⅓	⅓	½	½	½	½	⅔	⅔	¾

Directions: Steam asparagus and Brussels sprouts. Steam and mash the sweet potato. Next, add the walnut oil and pumpkin seeds to the sweet potato. Wrap the chicken in foil and bake in the oven at 350°F for 30 minutes or until done. Serve together. Enjoy!

Turkey Surprise

Ingredients	1200	1400	1600	1800	2000	2200	2400	2600	2800
Soy sauce (tbsp)	1	1¼	1⅓	1½	1⅔	1¾	2	2¼	2⅓
Cooked brown rice (cup)	⅛	⅛	¼	¼	¼	¼	⅓	⅓	⅓
Turkey breast (grams/oz.)	63/2.2	73.5/2.6	84/3	94.5/3.3	105/3.7	115.5/4	126/4.4	126/4.4	147/5
Extra-virgin olive oil (tbsp)	½	1	1	1	1	1	1	1	1
Spinach (cup)	¼	¼	¼	⅓	⅓	½	½	½	½

Directions: Sprinkle soy sauce over cooked brown rice. In a skillet, cook turkey breast with ½ tsp of olive oil. Place cooked turkey breast on top of a bed of spinach and serve with brown rice and soy sauce. Enjoy!

AFTERNOON SNACKS

Shake 'n Snack

Ingredients	1200	1400	1600	1800	2000	2200	2400	2600	2800
Whey protein powder (tbsp)	2	2½	3	3	3½	4	4	4	5
Spring water (cup)	½	½	⅔	¾	¾	1	1	1⅛	1⅛
Apples, diced (cup)	¼	¼	⅓	⅓	½	½	½	½	½
Almond(s)	3	3	3	4	4	5	5	5	6
Pumpkin seeds (cup)	⅛	⅛	⅛	⅛	⅛	⅛	⅛	⅛	⅛

Directions: In a shaker cup, mix whey protein powder with water. In a separate bowl, mix apples, almond(s), and pumpkin seeds together. Enjoy!

Nachos and Dip

Ingredients	1200	1400	1600	1800	2000	2200	2400	2600	2800
Low-fat baked tortilla chips	6	7	8	9	10	11	12	13	14
Low-fat Colby cheese, shredded (cup)	⅛	⅛	⅛	⅛	⅛	⅛	⅛	¼	¼
Nonfat Mozzarella cheese, shredded (cup)	¼	¼	¼	⅓	⅓	⅓	½	½	½
Guacamole (tbsp)	½	½	½	½	½	½	1	1	1
Salsa (cup)	½	½	⅔	¾	¾	¾	1	1⅛	1⅛

Directions: Place tortilla chips on a plate. Top with shredded cheese and microwave for about 35 seconds or until cheese is melted. Use guacamole and salsa as a dip. Enjoy!

Kiwi Energizer

Ingredients	1200	1400	1600	1800	2000	2200	2400	2600	2800
Banana, sliced (cup)	½	½	½	⅔	⅔	¾	¾	1	1
Flaxseed oil (tbsp)	⅓	½	½	½	⅔	⅔	¾	¾	1
Kiwi, sliced	1	1	1	1	1	1	1	1	1
Spring water (tbsp)	½	½	⅔	¾	¾	1	1	1¼	1¼
Whey protein powder (tbsp)	2	3	3	3	4	4	4½	5	5

Directions: In blender, combine banana, kiwi, and water, and blend well. Add whey protein powder and flaxseed and blend for additional 10 seconds. Enjoy!

Hummus and Veggies

Ingredients	1200	1400	1600	1800	2000	2200	2400	2600	2800
Cauliflower florets	6	7	8	9	10	11	12	13	14
Yellow pepper, sliced (cup)	1	1	1	1	1	1	1	1½	1½
Soy cheddar cheese (slices)	2	2½	3	3	3½	4	4½	5	5
Hummus (tbsp)	1	1	1	1	1	1½	1½	2	2

Directions: Dip cauliflower florets, peppers, and cheese into the hummus. Enjoy!

Crackers and Cheese

Ingredients	1200	1400	1600	1800	2000	2200	2400	2600	2800
Low-fat Swiss cheese slice(s)	1	1½	2	2	2	2	2½	3	3
Whole-wheat crackers	5	6	7	8	9	10	10	11	12

Directions: Place cheese on crackers. Enjoy!

Blueberry Yogurt

Ingredients	1200	1400	1600	1800	2000	2200	2400	2600	2800
Blueberries (cup)	⅛	⅛	⅛	⅛	⅛	¼	¼	¼	¼
Ground flaxseeds (tbsp)	½	½	½	⅔	¾	¾	¾	1	1
Plain low-fat yogurt (cup)	⅔	¾	¾	1	1	1⅛	1¼	1⅓	1½

Directions: Add blueberries and ground flaxseeds to yogurt. Enjoy!

Fruity Snack

Ingredients	1200	1400	1600	1800	2000	2200	2400	2600	2800
Blueberries (cup)	⅛	⅛	⅛	⅛	⅛	⅛	⅛	⅛	⅛
Kiwi	½	½	½	½	½	½	½	½	½
Ground flaxseed (tbsp)	⅔	¾	¾	1	1	1⅛	1¼	1⅓	1½
Strawberry (small)	1	1	1	1	1	1	1	1	1
Plain low-fat yogurt (cup)	¾	¾	1	1⅛	1⅛	1¼	1½	1½	1⅔

Directions: Stir fruit and flaxseed into the yogurt and enjoy!

Nutty Bread

Ingredients	1200	1400	1600	1800	2000	2200	2400	2600	2800
Almond butter (tbsp)	⅛	⅛	⅛	⅛	⅛	⅛	⅛	⅛	⅛
Whole-grain bread (slices)	2	2	3	3	3	4	4	4	5
Soy nuts (cup)	¼	¼	¼	⅓	⅓	⅓	½	½	½

Directions: Spread almond butter on bread and enjoy with soy nuts.

EXERCISING THE DEMONS

MINDSET

With every workout I am losing fat, increasing lean muscle tissue, and enhancing my mobility and energy.

In order for you to succeed in transforming your body and achieving your health improvement, muscle building, or fat loss goal, you must focus on three necessary components: the correct mindset, proper nutrition, and a fitness program specifically designed with the end result in mind. Any "weight loss" program that is missing one (or more) of these components is fundamentally flawed and doomed to failure. In particular, if you are looking at a program that does not advocate exercise, do not even consider it. Moreover, if the program does not include weight training, you will lose muscle mass, which, as discussed, is the last thing you want to do.

There are countless benefits to a regular exercise program, including improved circulation, enhanced mood, the burning of body fat, the maintenance and building of lean muscle tissue, as well as a reduction in the risk of stroke and development of diseases such as Alzheimer's, diabetes, and cancer.

The inclusion of resistance training in your workout regime extends a lesser-known benefit for both men and women: Strong muscles are attached to strong bones.

In addition to gaining muscular strength, people who regularly train with weights will also develop stronger bones. In a study conducted at Tufts University and published in the *Journal of the American Medical Association*, researchers looked at the effects of strength training on postmenopausal women. Over the course of a 12-month period, participants demonstrated dramatic improvements in hip and spine bone density, strength, and balance.

Working to become stronger is important since the amount of weight lifted is related to improvements in total body bone mass density (BMD). There is strong evidence to support a linear relationship between BMD change and total exercise-specific weight lifted.

Women should not be afraid of challenging their muscles with progressive resistance. As you know, it is essential to train with resistance in order to build lean muscle tissue and increase your metabolic rate. In order to increase lean muscle, you must subject your muscles to adequate resistance or stress in order to elicit muscular hypertrophy or growth. When we exercise with the goal of increasing lean muscle, we are putting stress on the bones, which will cause them to grow stronger in response to this stress.

The message is clear: If you are serious about changing your body composition, improving your health, and developing a more positive mental state, then it is time that you became serious about your exercise program.

COMMON EXERCISE MYTHS

Before you begin your exercise program, it is important to dispel any myths that are holding you back from developing the perfect exercise program and getting into great shape.

Most of the following myths have been around for so many years that they have been universally accepted, and one of the biggest challenges I face is convincing people that what they held to be true is in fact completely false. Over the years I have compiled a list of the 10 most common myths when it comes to exercise.

1. Strength Training Will Make Women Bulky

Many women are afraid that strength training will make them overly muscular; they believe the notion that strength training is only for men. This is untrue. In fact, women do not have to worry about looking like a bodybuilder simply because women don't have enough testosterone to create big, bulky muscles. To become a bodybuilder, a woman would have to inject exogenous hormones and dramatically change her training program to reflect this goal.

The truth is that strength training has enormous benefits for women. In a recent study, sedentary postmenopausal women were randomly assigned to do strength-training exercises twice a week or to do no additional exercise. After a year, the strength-trainers had greater bone density, muscle mass, muscle strength, balance, and less body fat than the sedentary women.

Women have less bone and muscle than men and therefore need to take care of what they've got. This is the reason why women are at greater risk of osteoporosis than men. Loss of muscle also puts women at an increased risk of disability as they age. Strength training will help with both of these issues.

2. Certain Exercises Are Great for "Spot" Reducing

One commonly held myth is that if people exercise one area, it will cause fat to be removed from that area. In gyms around the country you will find countless people trying to lose midsection fat by performing hundreds upon thousands of repetitions on abdominal machines. The same can be said for hip and thigh devices—every day scores of women are burning their way through multiple sets in an attempt to spot reduce body fat. However, spot-reducing exercise is a myth. Abdominal and hip exercises can strengthen and tone muscles, but those muscles are hidden underneath the subcutaneous layer of fat. Losing fat pounds through proper nutrition and exercise will get rid of excess flab; however, where you first lose the fat depends on your genes. Some folks are simply more resistant to losing fat in certain areas than others. However, in most cases (especially with women) losing fat around the waist is easier than losing it at the hips. Keep in mind that if your goal is to lose fat in a particular area, then your *overall* body fat must be reduced.

However, the concept of spot reduction does hold some promise, not through targeted exercise but rather through targeted supplementation. Renowned strength coach and exercise physiologist Charles Poliquin has developed a testing system known as Biosignature Modulation. This system looks at the amount of fat a person carries in specific sites of the body and correlates this to a site-specific supplementation protocol. According to Charles, those individuals who have a high amount of body fat in the umbilical region (belly fat) are often found to suffer from chronically elevated cortisol levels. For these people, the supplement phosphatydylserine (found in green drinks) has been shown to reduce circulating cortisol, as well as improve mood and immunity and alleviate depression. Fish oils are also recommended for regulating cortisol and the associated umbilical fat deposition. For those holding fat in the "love handle" region, fish oils as well as flaxseeds are effective due to their ability to control blood sugar levels and insulin. This is a new area of research and is showing lots of promise. For more information, please visit www.charlespoliquin.com.

3. Exercise Burns Lots of Calories

People have the mistaken idea that exercise burns lots of calories; however, the truth is that many of the exercises people do burn very few calories! For example, depending on the person, walking or running a mile burns about 100 calories, but sitting still for the same time burns about 50 or 60 calories. That doesn't mean you should give up on exercise. The more you exercise, the more fit you'll become, and the more fit you are, the more calories you burn *all the time*. That means you'll not only burn more calories when exercising (because you can walk more briskly or work out with greater intensity), but also that your body will burn more fat for energy because your muscles will become more adept at using an enzyme that oxidizes fat. People who exercise less burn more carbohydrates instead.

People who follow the Fat-Fighter Diet program and exercise while eating the correct foods at the right times also lose less lean body mass (muscle) than those dieters who just cut calories. In addition, ongoing physical activity will help with the toughest problem of all—keeping fat off. Studies have shown that after people lose fat, one of the best predictors of maintaining the fat loss is whether they exercise regularly.

4. If You Don't Lose Weight, There's No Point in Exercising

While a desire to lose fat is what gets most people off the couch and into their walking shoes, the positive impact goes far beyond the visible changes that accompany regular exercise.

Regular exercise, among many other wonderful benefits, lowers the risk of diabetes and heart disease, improves blood-clotting mechanisms, lowers triglycerides, and raises HDL ("good" cholesterol) levels. It improves sleep and relieves both depression and anxiety. Studies have shown that a single 30-minute exercise session will improve mood and feelings of well-being. Regular exercise is also excellent for relieving stress and may even raise levels of serotonin, the "feel good" brain neurotransmitter.

5. You Cannot Be Fit with Fat

There is a misconception that all people with higher-than-average body fat percentages are sedentary, unfit, and at high risk of disease. Healthy bodies can come in all shapes and sizes. What is important is activity. Motivating all of those unfit people—fat or thin—to increase physical activity could make a difference in lowering risk factors like high cholesterol, high blood pressure, and diabetes. Yet doctors rarely test a patient's fitness as part of a checkup.

Fitness is an important predictor of mortality, and it is inexcusable not to evaluate it as part of a person's health risk. It is also nearly impossible to evaluate at a glance.

6. No Pain, No Gain

Many people still believe that in order to receive any benefit from exercise, they have to work at a very high-intensity level. However, moderate-intensity exercise lowers health risks just as much as high-intensity exercise. The trick is making sure that the exercise is at least equivalent to walking at a pace of 3–4 miles an hour.

Running or jogging is, by definition, high intensity. But walking, raking leaves, and mowing lawns may be either moderate or low intensity.

When your goal is to change the composition of your body, it is important to vary the intensity of your strength training and cardio workouts. Periodizing your training program (by including periods of low-, moderate-, and high-intensity training phases) will produce far better results than using a workout with the same level of intensity all the time. The Fat-Fighter Diet includes a great periodized training program for you to try in Chapter16.

7. If You Cannot Exercise Regularly, Don't Bother

It takes 10–12 weeks of regular exercise to become what is commonly known as "fit"—that is, to improve your performance on a general endurance or V02 max test (a test that measures oxygen consumption during intense exercise), but your health can improve after that first brisk walk or run. For example, take a 50-year-old man who is somewhat overweight and typically has moderately elevated blood sugar, triglycerides, or blood pressure. After only one exercise session of moderate intensity such as 30–40 minutes of brisk walking, those numbers will be reduced.

And improvements happen not just while you exercise. If you exercise at five o'clock in the afternoon, the improvement will be there the next morning.

Everyone should try to get at least 30 minutes of moderate activity on most or preferably all days of the week. But if you can't, don't let that stop you from taking a short walk around the block or even around the local mall because even a small amount of exercise has benefits.

8. If You Did Not Exercise When You Were Younger, It Would Be Dangerous to Start When You Are Older

Many people think they're too old to start an exercise program. Often they think it's unsafe because they have heart disease or diabetes or because they're too out of shape to start.

The truth is you are never too old to start. In one study, nursing-home residents whose ages ranged from 72–98 did just 10 weeks of strength training. All participants improved their muscle strength, ability to climb stairs, and walking speed!

The same goes for people with chronic diseases. People with arthritis often say they cannot exercise, but some of the greatest examples of exercise benefits are found in people with arthritis. This is because exercise reduces pain and increases range of motion, strength, and mobility.

The trick here is to start with easy exercise and work your way up to more vigorous exercise. There can be risks involved with starting a brand new exercise program, and it is very important to visit your doctor to get the go-ahead before you begin. Your doctor can help you to make careful choices about the amount and type of exercise you introduce your body to in the early stages. In a recent study, inactive people—especially men who had high cholesterol, angina, were smokers, or were obese—were 10 times more likely to have a heart attack within an hour of exerting themselves (usually by jogging or heavy lifting) than at other times. Before beginning the exercise portion of this book, please take the time to complete the Par-Q Questionnaire on page 145-146 and check with your doctor if you answer "yes" to any of the questions.

9. Aerobics Is Best for Body Shaping and Fat Loss

This is a widespread myth throughout the entire fitness community: Weights are just for building huge muscles and aerobics are for burning fat. The truth is that weight training is *by far* the best exercise for long-term fat loss and strength gain. While different types of aerobic training in the form of running, jogging, etc., are all great, they should be done as an adjunct to a properly designed resistance-training program. This, in combination with a good stretching program, will produce lifelong lasting changes to your body composition.

10. Weight Gain Is Inevitable as You Age

Most people get fatter as they get older, but they don't have to. It is a matter of reduced physical activity levels and lower metabolic rate caused by a loss of lean body mass (muscle).

This lifelong loss of lean body mass reduces our base metabolic rate as we age. This subtle change occurs between ages 20 and 30. As the percentage of body fat gradually increases, it produces an ever-decreasing calorie requirement. And this lower metabolic rate means that unless you eat less, you'll gain weight over time. However, exercise can mount a two-pronged defense against middle-age spread and muscle loss. Any activity makes you burn more calories, so you're less likely to wind up with an excess, and strength training can offset the loss of muscle mass.

Beginning at age 40 in women and at 60 in men, we lose 6–8 percent of our muscle per decade. However, after only two months of strength training, women can recover a decade of loss and men can recover two decades!

That's with only three weekly sessions that take about 40–50 minutes each, including warm-up, rest periods, and stretching. The actual time required to perform the exercises that increase muscle mass is very insignificant compared to the return you will receive on your investment.

ACTION

Banish these myths from your belief system. Replace them with the belief and conviction that you can and will achieve your goal.

THE NECESSARY COMPONENTS
OF AN EFFECTIVE WORKOUT 15

Perhaps the world's most famous fitness icon, Arnold Schwarzenegger, describes fitness as being "the development of all the body's physical capabilities." These capabilities include all of the following:

- *Aerobic conditioning or cardio:* This is any activity that utilizes a vast amount of oxygen, which is delivered to the muscles by the lungs, heart, and circulatory system. Various activities are useful in developing this conditioning, including running, sprinting, cycling, skiing, circuit training, and jumping rope.
- *Muscular conditioning:* Resistance or weight training is the single best method to develop and strengthen the muscles. This is done by working the muscles through a full range of motion with a focus on both the eccentric (lowering) and concentric (raising) portions of a given movement.
- *Flexibility:* Stretching the muscles, tendons, and ligaments surrounding the joints of your body will promote increased range of motion, decrease the chance of injury, and improve recovery between workouts.

PAR-Q QUESTIONNAIRE

Before we begin the fitness component of the Fat-Fighter Diet, it is important that you complete the following Par-Q questionnaire.

If you are between the ages of 15 and 69, this test will tell you whether or not you should check with your doctor before you start exercising. If you are over 69 years of age, and you are not accustomed to being very active, check with your doctor before beginning your exercise routine.

Please read these questions carefully and answer each one honestly with yes or no.

· *Has your doctor ever said that you have a heart condition and that you should do only physical activity recommended by a doctor?*
· *Do you feel pain in your chest when you do physical activity?*
· *In the past month, have you had chest pain when you were not doing physical activity?*
· *Do you lose your balance because of dizziness or do you ever lose consciousness?*
· *Do you have a bone or joint problem (for example, back, knee, or hip) that could be worsened by a change in your physical activity?*
· *Is your doctor currently prescribing drugs (for example, water pills) for your blood pressure or heart condition?*
· *Do you know of any other reason why you should not do physical activity?*

If you answered:

Yes to one or more questions, talk to your doctor before you start becoming more physically active and before you complete the fitness testing. Tell your doctor about this questionnaire and which questions to which you answered yes.

No to all questions, you can be reasonably sure that you can take part in the following fitness testing and start becoming more physically active. It is recommended that you have your blood pressure tested. If you have a reading over 144/94, talk with your doctor before you start any fitness program.

COMPONENT 1: AEROBIC CONDITIONING

If you are like most of my clients, one of your main goals is to burn body fat. In order to accomplish this, you must create a calorie deficit. This means that you burn more calories than you consume. This is done in two ways:

1. By reducing calorie intake from food (but not so drastically so as to induce your body's starvation response and slow your metabolism as discussed in Chapter 1.
2. By performing regular exercise to build muscle and burn calories.

With a properly designed lifestyle-focused program like this one, both methods are used. Cardiovascular exercise plays an important part in your fat loss quest. In addition to improving heart and lung capacity, cardio will also increase your metabolic rate as well as fat-burning enzymes and hormones. Cardio is also a great way to burn extra calories.

In this section you will learn everything you need to know about what type and how much cardio you need to do in order to achieve your goals. Don't waste this information! Once you have discovered your personalized routine, revisit your goals and update them to reflect your new knowledge. Take a moment to schedule in your weekly cardio training sessions. Map out exactly when, where, and how much you are going to do and stick to your plan. Decide on how you will fit it in with your resistance-training routine (more on that to come) and go for it!

Approved Cardiovascular Exercise

When I am training a client one on one, I often have them to do some homework on their off days from the gym. Usually I ask them to perform some cardiovascular exercise at least two or three days per week. When I check to see what they have been up to, I hear some interesting definitions for cardio such as gardening, strolling, doing chores, and (my personal favorite) playing golf. Don't get me wrong, these are all excellent, healthy activities. However, these activities are not the best choices when you are trying to make a change to your body fat percentage. These activities are recreational rather than fitness promoting. They are too low intensity to produce any real result. Moderate- to high-intensity cardiovascular exercise is required if your goal is to change the shape of your body and burn body fat. Some good cardiovascular activities to consider are: brisk walking, sprinting, stair-climbing, obstacle course training, kickboxing, stationary bike, elliptical trainer, and treadmill.

What Is the Right Amount of Cardio for Me?

The right amount of cardio for you will depend upon your goal.

Healthy lifestyle: If your goal is to develop and maintain a healthy lifestyle, dedicate yourself to 20–30 minutes of moderate cardio activities two or three times per week.

Fat loss: If your goal is to lose body fat, increasing this to 30–40 minutes of moderate to high cardio three to five days per week (30 minutes if you are performing cardio on an empty stomach immediately upon waking and 40 minutes if it is done at any other time). For a more extreme result, you may want to increase this to once per day. However, this should never be done for more than two weeks and is reserved only for those who want to reach a low single-digit body fat percentage.

Increase lean muscle and strength: If your goal is to increase your lean muscle tissue and grow stronger, do a *maximum* of 30–40 minutes of cardio, two or three days per week. (Your body requires more calories to build new muscle tissue. Doing too much cardio while trying to build muscle can be counterproductive.)

The Fitness Test

A fitness test is a great way to determine what type of physical shape you are in.

If you feel pain while performing any of the proceeding test exercises, please stop and consult your physician or a certified fitness professional.

1. *How long have you been engaged in a consistent resistance-training program?*
   Less than six months: score 1
   Six months to one year: score 2
   More than one year: score 3

2. *How many times per week do you perform cardiovascular exercise, e.g., walking, running, stair climber, etc.?*
   Once per week: score 1
   Two to four times per week: score 2
   Five or more times per week: score 3

3. *How would you rate the intensity of your average cardio session?*
   Low: score 1
   Medium: score 2
   High: score 3

4. *How long can you hold this position? (Plank test)*
   0–30 seconds: score 1
   31–60 seconds: score 2
   61 seconds or more: score 3

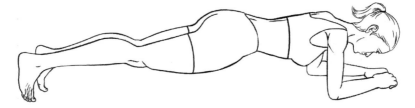

5. *How long can you hold this position? (Side plank test)*

    0–30 seconds: score 1

    31–60 seconds: score 2

    61 seconds or more: score 3

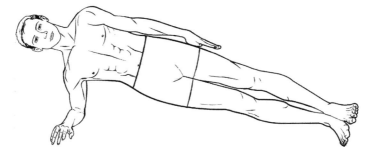

6. *How many abdominal crunches can you perform?*

    Less than 10: score 1

    10–20: score 2

    20–30: score 3

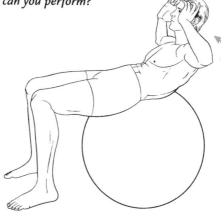

7. *How many push-ups can you perform? (Modified for women; full body for men)*

    Less than 5: score 1

    5–15: score 2

    15 or more: score 3

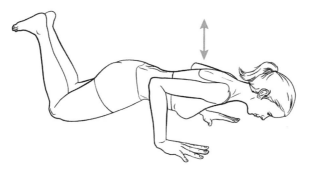

8. *How many squats can you perform? (With or without dumbells squat down until thighs are parallel to the floor.)*

> *Less than 10:* score 1
> *10–20:* score 2
> *20 or more:* score 3

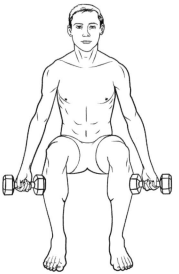

Interpreting Your Results

Add up all of your scores from each of the tests. Use the scale below to see how you did:

8–13 = Beginner

The beginning—what a great place to start! Congratulations on making the decision to begin this journey. Follow your diet and exercise program and soon you will be seeing (and feeling) the results of your efforts.

14–20 = Intermediate

Good for you! You are well on your way to building your best body inside and out! Keep up with your exercise program and be sure to do regular cardio workouts in addition to resistance training for optimal results.

21–24 = Advanced

Give yourself a pat on the back, you old pro! Clearly your exercise program has done wonders for you. To keep the results coming, be sure to change it every four to six weeks. Periodizing your program is needed to take it to the next level.

What Is the Right Intensity Level for Me?

Now you know how much cardio to do, but what is the correct intensity level for you? This will depend on your current level of fitness. Performing your cardio using the correct target heart rate (THR) for your body and goal is important to your success. To ensure accuracy and safety, especially for beginners, I recommend that you purchase a heart-rate monitor. You can find wristwatch-type monitors at most fitness equipment stores. Your THR is calculated as follows:

(220 – your age) – resting heart rate (RHR) × intensity % + RHR. Sound confusing? Don't worry, I'll walk you through it!

Use this scale to determine your intensity level:

Beginner: 50–65 percent intensity
Intermediate: 65–80 percent intensity
Advanced: 80–90 percent intensity

Now let's plug in the numbers to see how this works.

> Example: Jane Doe
> *Age:* 35
> *RHR:* 75
> *Experience:* Beginner (50–65 percent intensity)
> 220 – 35 (her age) = 185
> 185 – 75 (resting heart rate) = 110
> 110 × .50 (lower end of intensity level) = 55
> 55 + 75 (resting heart rate) = 130
> Therefore, the lower end of her target range is 130. To find her higher end, the same equation is repeated using .65 as the intensity level.
> Target heart rate = 130–146 beats per minute

Change is Good

Performing your cardiovascular exercise in your target heart rate zone will produce fantastic results. Be sure to monitor your heart rate for the duration of your cardio session (using a heart rate monitor, which is more accurate than trying to check it manually while exercising). However, like resistance training, the duration, type, intensity, and frequency of your cardiovascular workouts must change every couple of weeks in order to avoid your body's inevitable adaptation response. Here are some changes to consider:

1. Interval training: Try varying the intensity within a given workout by incorporating periods of high-, medium- and low-intensity intervals. High-intensity interval training or HIIT has been shown to be a superior way to perform cardiovascular exercise for fat loss. With HIIT training, you combine short intervals (15–30 seconds) of moderate intensity (60 percent) with longer intervals (90 seconds) of high-intensity (75–85 percent) followed by a brief low-intensity (50 percent) recovery period before repeating.

   Note: Due to the high intensity of HIIT training, only use this method once you have developed a good base of cardiovascular conditioning. The duration of a HIIT cardio training workout should not exceed 30 minutes, including warm-up and cooldown.
2. Substitute one form of cardiovascular exercise for another, i.e., stair climbing for running, or swimming for walking.
3. Vary the duration of your cardio workout. If you have been doing 20 minutes, try 30.
4. Change the frequency of your cardiovascular workouts. Instead of twice per week, try three times per week.

ACTION

Do this calculation yourself in order to know your target heart rate. Be sure to change your cardiovascular exercise every few weeks in order to keep results coming.

Timing is Everything

When it comes to your cardio, the time of day that you exercise can depend on what you are trying to accomplish.

If your goal is to improve general health or increase lean muscle, your cardio should be performed whenever it suits you best. Just remember to make it a priority and schedule it in; otherwise you may *forget* to do it!

However, if your goal is fat loss, do your cardio first thing in the morning on an empty stomach. Research studies have shown that fat is burned up to 300 percent faster when you exercise first thing in the morning compared to exercising later in the day! One such study, conducted at Kansas State University and published in *Medicine and Science in Sports and Exercise,* proved that body fat is burned faster when exercise is done in the fasted state in the morning than when it's done later in the day. Early morning cardio is best for fat loss for a number of reasons:

1. Because you have spent the previous eight to 12 hours sleeping—essentially a mini-fast—your body's glycogen stores and blood glucose levels are low, enabling you to access more fat for energy.
2. Performing your cardio first thing in the morning will elevate your metabolism for several hours after your workout.
3. You are more likely to forgo cardio after you come home from a long day at work. Doing your cardio first thing in the morning ensures that it gets done and boosts your mood-enhancing endorphins for the day.

Early Mornings Not for You?

If doing cardio first thing in the morning is not possible and you are forced to combine cardiovascular and resistance-training workouts, do your cardio after your weights. Doing so will ensure that you have sufficient energy for your resistance training and will enhance the fat-burning effect of cardio due to the reduction of your body's glycogen and glucose levels, thus making fat the primary fuel source.

ACTION
Schedule your cardiovascular workouts and practise consistency for continual progress. Make this a habit.

COMPONENT 2: MUSCULAR CONDITIONING

Improving your muscular conditioning using resistance training is the second vital component to long-term health, fitness, and fat loss. In addition to your cardiovascular workouts, you must perform resistance training to build muscle and increase your metabolic rate. This combination of aerobics *plus* resistance training (and flexibility) will result in permanent and lifelong changes to your body composition and health. I have made this easy for you to follow by including detailed workout routines that show you exactly how much, how often, and what you should do in order to achieve your goal.

Planning Ahead

The human body is a highly adaptable machine. As human beings, we have the ability to adapt and become accustomed to almost any environment and stimulus. And so it is when it comes to your workouts. Those of you who have prior exercise experience may have noticed that after a certain amount of time, your workouts just seem to stop producing results. Worse still, you may find yourself regressing and actually losing muscle definition and strength. This is because your body has adapted to your workout routine. In order to avoid this and achieve continual results month after month, year after year, you must periodize your training program.

What Is Periodization?

Periodization is the process of varying a training program at regular time intervals to optimize gains in all areas of physical performance. This is accomplished through the use of various phases of training, both in the short term and in the long term. Some proven benefits of periodization are improved strength, muscular endurance, and muscle development. Periodization will maximize results in a minimal amount of time! (The Fat-Fighter Diet will introduce you to the first phase of periodization for your Fat Loss, Healthy Lifestyle, and Increase Lean Muscle and Strength workouts. Subsequent phases can be found using our Web training tool at www.ebodi.com).

Choosing Your Resistance-Training Workout

First of all, congratulations on making it this far. You are clearly committed to making the changes and doing the work necessary to succeed. I have designed your exercise program so that it can be done at home using minimal equipment. The only equipment you will need to complete your workouts are dumbbells (preferably 5–30 lbs) and a stability ball that fits your body.

Using free weights engages more core muscles during the execution of an exercise, resulting in increased coordination, mobility, strength, power, and fat loss.

Fat Loss, Healthy Lifestyle, and Increase Lean Muscle and Strength Workouts

The next step is to determine what type of resistance-training workout is best suited to achieving your fitness goal. The Fat-Fighter Diet features three distinct workout streams: Fat Loss, Healthy Lifestyle, and Increase Lean Muscle and Strength.

Fat Loss Stream

This stream is focused on body fat reduction using the proper mix of resistance training and aerobics. This stream uses short rest intervals and a unique and innovative progression of the circuit training method. *This is an extremely effective exercise program for fat loss.*

Healthy Lifestyle Stream

This phase deals with functional training and follows the flexibility-stability-strength-power continuum. All of these components are worked within this stream, which places a strong emphasis on improving the four primal movement patterns of the human body.

Four Primal Movement Patterns

There are four pillars of human movement: lunge, squat, push/pull, and rotation. These primal movement patterns are progressed using various training modalities.

This phase would be suitable for the beginner, the active person, and the "weekend warrior" alike. This stream will ensure a stable, functionally strong body for life.

Increase Lean Muscle and Strength Stream

This stream is perfect for those individuals who are focused on developing their muscle and strength to the fullest. Various techniques will be used within this stream. The workouts will increase muscle hypertrophy (growth) as well as strength.

ACTION
Determine the appropriate starting point for your fitness and experience level. Next, choose the workout that corresponds with your fitness level and goal.

COMPONENT 3: FLEXIBILITY

Stretching is the most neglected component of most people's workout. The stretching of your muscles, tendons, ligaments, and joint structures is vital for promoting and improving range of motion and will also improve the overall look of your body.

Why Be Flexible?

There are many benefits to a good flexibility program:

1. *Improving Physical Performance.* A flexible joint structure has greater range of motion than an inflexible structure. This improved range of motion allows for greater muscle recruitment and increased strength and performance.
2. *Decreasing Chance of Injury.* By increasing your range of motion you are less

likely to become injured by exceeding the range of your muscle tissues and ligaments during activity.

3. *Improved Posture.* Inactive lifestyles and poor postural habits can contribute to muscular imbalances and inflexibility. Stretching will help keep your soft tissue structures in alignment, making it easier for you to maintain good posture.

4. *Reduced Muscle Soreness.* Pre- and post-workout stretching helps to reduce the muscle soreness often experienced with exercising.

5. *Reduces the Risk of Lower Back Pain.* Lower back pain is one of the top listed ailments in North America. Because stretching promotes muscular relaxation, it will also aid in the reduction of lower back pain. Maintaining flexibility in the hamstrings, hip flexors, quadriceps, and other muscles attached to the pelvis will reduces stress to the lower back.

6. *Increases Blood Flow.* Stretching increases blood supply to the joint structures. The increased blood flow results in an increase in tissue temperature as well as circulation and the transportation of nutrients. Stretching will also increase the production of joint synovial fluid, which lubricates and transports nutrients to the joints' cartilage. This will in turn increase range of motion and reduce joint degeneration.

7. *Encourages a Peaceful Mind and Body.* Flexibility training not only decreases muscle soreness and increases performance, it also relaxes both mind and body. Stretching will improve your overall sense of well-being, while also increasing your feelings of satisfaction and gratitude.

Many people neglect this area of their physical fitness. Do not be one of them! Flexibility is a vital component to a well-balanced exercise program and produces benefits that cannot be achieved by any other exercise or activity.

ACTION
Perform each of the pre- and post-workout stretches on the days that you are exercising.

THE RESISTANCE-TRAINING WORKOUTS

All of the proceeding workouts can be performed in less than 60 minutes. Avoid training for longer as cortisol rises sharply after 45–60 minutes of strength training. To begin, simply choose the workout stream you would like to start with and begin at your appropriate level (beginner, intermediate, or advanced). Remember that you should stay in each level for four weeks before proceeding to the next level. You can jump between streams, but be sure to always work at the right fitness level for you.

Before You Begin

Before you begin each resistance-training session, be sure to warm up for five minutes with some light cardiovascular activity such as stationary bike riding or treadmill. Following this warm-up, perform each of the pre-workout stretches as shown in the flexibility exercise section (pages 183–85). Study each of the exercises and carefully read each instruction to ensure proper form and safety.

After Each Workout

Be sure to finish each workout with your post-workout stretching routine.

Breathing

While breathing comes naturally to us, there is a preferred method to breathing while performing resistance-training exercise. The first point to remember is to not hold your breath. Concentrate on inhaling deeply with each eccentric (lowering) portion of the exercise and exhaling upon the concentric (raising) portion. Breathe in deeply through your nose and exhale through your mouth. When performing cardio, be sure to focus on bringing air deep into your lungs and avoid shallow gasping, which may indicate that you are working at too high an intensity for your fitness level.

Scheduling Your Workouts

The Fat-Fighter Diet asks that you perform resistance training on three nonconsecutive days each week. For maximum results, you are also required to perform cardiovascular exercise two to five days per week. Your goal should be to perform physical activity five or six days per week, with three bouts of resistance training and two or three cardio sessions. Your schedule may appear as follows:

- Monday: resistance
- Tuesday: cardio
- Wednesday: resistance
- Thursday: cardio
- Friday: resistance
- Saturday: cardio
- Sunday: rest

This is optimal. If you find yourself short on time for a particular week, you can combine your resistance training and cardio on the same day (resistance training to be completed first, followed by cardio). However, this is not optimal. Performing your resistance training and cardiovascular workouts on alternate days will produce the best results.

Now, let's get started!

EXERCISE GUIDE

CORE-STRENGTHENING EXERCISES

Your core muscles are the foundational muscles of your midsection that you cannot see. To activate your core, pull your lower abdominal muscles inward toward your spine and squeeze your gluteus muscles.

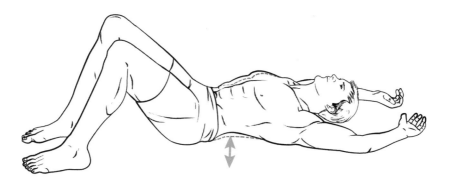

Pelvic Tilt

Starting Point: Lie on your back with knees bent, feet flat on the floor, and arms resting over your head. Activate your core.

Movement: Perform a slight posterior pelvic tilt (flatten your lower back against the floor). Hold for the recommended time.

Key Points: Maintain your core activation. Do not let your neck hyper-extend or chin jut forward. Your upper body should remain motionless.

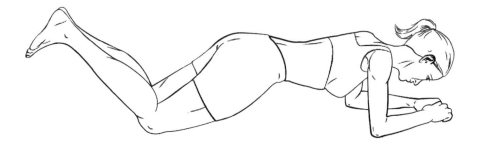

Front Plank (on your knees)

Starting Point: Begin in a prone position, with elbows bent and fists closed and positioned under your shoulders. Activate your core.

Movement: Lift your body onto your forearms and knees. Maintain your core activation and hold for the recommended time.

Key Points: Your spine should maintain a neutral position at all times. The gluteus should remain activated throughout the duration of exercise. Keep your chin tucked in.

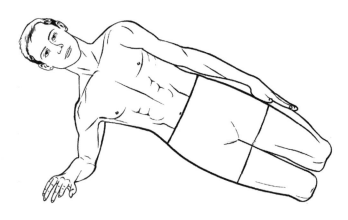

Side Plank (on your knees)

Starting Point: Lie on your side with knees bent. Activate your core. Place an elbow directly under your shoulder for support.

Movement: Maintain your core activation, lift your body up onto your forearm, and hold for the recommended time. Repeat for the opposite side.

Key Points: Your head must stay in a neutral position. Keep your spine in a straight line and don't allow your hips to droop toward the floor. Your core must be activated for the duration of the exercise.

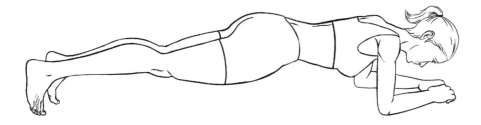

Front Plank (on toes)

Starting Point: Starting in a prone position, bend your elbows and place your fists under your shoulders. Activate your core.

Movement: Lift your body onto your forearms and toes. Maintain your core activation and hold for the recommended time.

Key Points: Your spine should maintain a neutral position at all times. Keep your chin tucked in and don't allow your hips to droop toward the floor.

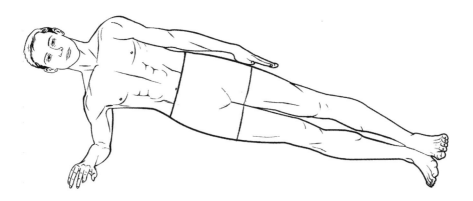

Side Plank (on toes)

Starting Point: Lie on your side with legs extended. Activate your core. Place your elbow directly under your shoulder for support.

Movement: Maintain your core activation and lift your body onto your forearm and outside edge of your foot and hold for

the recommended time. Keep your entire spine in a straight line and don't allow your hips to droop toward the floor. Repeat for the opposite side.

Key Points: Your head must stay in a neutral position. Your core must be activated for the duration of the exercise.

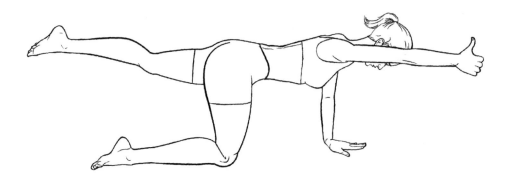

Quadruped (on knees)

Starting Point: Start on your hands and knees with your core activated.

Movement: Slowly raise one arm with the thumb up and the opposite leg until it is parallel to the floor. Hold for the recommended time and slowly lower your arm and leg to the ground while maintaining proper alignment. Repeat with the opposite side.

Key Points: Maintain your core activation and proper posture alignment. Think of lengthening your body as you raise your arm and leg rather than simply lifting.

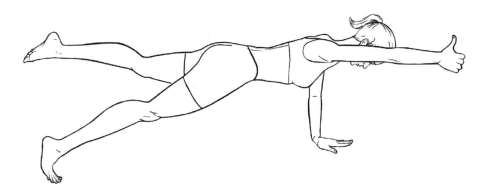

Quadruped

Starting Point: Start in a push-up position

Movement: Lift one arm (put thumb up) and the opposite leg. Keep both arm and leg straight while lifting arm up parallel to the floor. Hold for the recommended time.

Key Points: Maintain your core activation and proper posture alignment. Think of lengthening your body as you raise your arm and leg rather than simply lifting.

ABDOMINAL EXERCISES

Your abdominal muscles are the muscles of your stomach region (front and side).

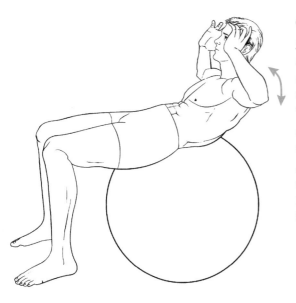

Crunch

Starting Point: Sit on an exercise ball, and activate your core. Slowly walk feet out and lie back on the ball. Your head and shoulders should be supported on the ball with the head slightly tilted back.

Movement: Slowly curl spine upward as far as you can comfortably control.

Key Points: Your chin should be tucked in toward your chest throughout the movement. Core activation should be maintained for the duration of the exercise.

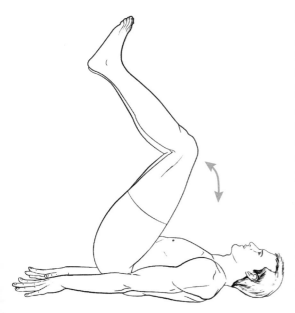

Reverse Crunch

Starting Point: Lie flat on your back with both knees bent, toes pointing straight ahead, and arms at the sides. Activate your core.

Movement: While maintaining core activation, curl your legs up until the knees are aligned with the hips. From this position, contract the lower abdominals and curl your lower body up. Hold for the recommended time and slowly lower to the starting position. Repeat for the recommended repetitions.

Key Points: Your chin should be tucked toward chest throughout the movement. Core activation should be maintained for the duration of the exercise.

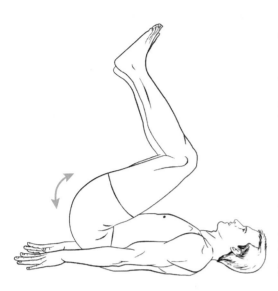

Knees Up

Starting Point: Lie flat on your back with both legs bent to 90 degrees, knees pointing straight up in the air, arms resting at your sides for support. Activate your core.

Movement: Raise both legs straight into the air so that hips are off the ground. Use only abdominal strength with no additional help from the arms. Hold for the recommended time and slowly lower back down to the ground.

Key Points: Keep your arms relaxed—do not push or help the movement with your arms. Maintain your core activation throughout the movement and raise your legs straight up and not toward your head.

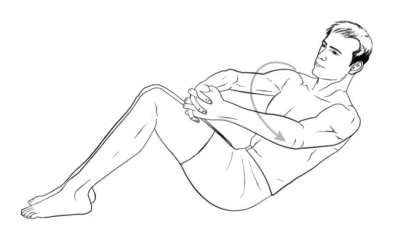

Russian Twist

Starting Point: Sit on the floor with both knees bent to 90 degrees and your feet flat. Lean your trunk back to a 45-degree angle and maintain a neutral spine. Activate your core.

Movement: Rotate your trunk from the center to the right side with arms outstretched parallel to your chest. Do the recommended repetitions and repeat with the opposite side.

Key Points: Maintain the trunk angle. Core activation should be held for the duration of the set. Keep your chin tucked throughout the movement. The movement should originate from the core/abdominals and not from the shoulders and arms.

THIGH STRENGTHENERS

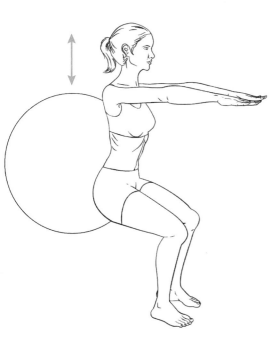

Ball Squat

Starting Point: Place a stability ball against the wall. Stand with both feet pointing straight ahead and gently lean back so that the lumbar curve is supported by the ball. Activate your core.

Movement: While maintaining core stability, descend slowly by bending at the knees and hips until thighs are parallel to the floor. Return to the starting position by driving through the feet and extending through ankle, knee, and hip joints while maintaining equal weight distribution on both feet.

Key Points: Maintain your core stability. Your knees should line up over the second and third toes.

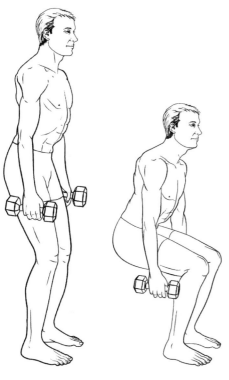

Dumbbell Squat

Starting Point: Stand with your feet pointing straight ahead while holding a dumbbell in each hand. Activate your core.

Movement: While maintaining core stability, descend slowly to parallel by bending at the knees and hips. Return to the starting position by driving through the feet and extending through ankle, knee, and hip joints while maintaining equal weight distribution on both feet.

Key Points: Maintain your core stability and your alignment (knees should line up over the second and third toes).

Front Lunge

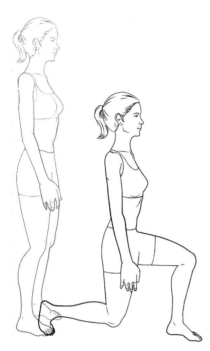

Starting Point: Stand with your feet shoulder-width apart and your arms hanging at the sides. Activate your core.

Movement: Lunge forward with one leg, landing on your heel then your forefoot. Lower your torso by flexing the knee and hip of the front leg. Extend the knee and hip of the forward leg and return to a standing position. Repeat for recommended repetitions and switch to the opposite leg.

Key Points: Maintain your core activation. Keep your torso upright during the movement.

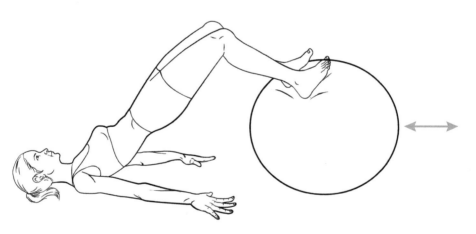

Hamstring Curl

Starting Point: Lie on the floor with hands at your sides, legs straight, and both heels positioned on the ball. Raise your buttocks off the floor. Activate your core.

Movement: Flex both knees and press up onto your heels while simultaneously rolling the ball inwards toward your buttocks.

Slowly return to the starting position by extending your knees. Repeat for the recommended repetitions.

Key Points: Maintain your core activation. Keep your torso stable. Avoid rolling off the sides of the ball.

CHEST STRENGTHENERS

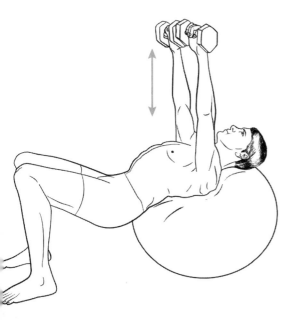

Incline Chest Press

Starting Point: Grasp two dumbbells and lie on the ball with your head and shoulders supported by the ball. Lower your hips below shoulder level and maintain this position. Activate your core.

Movement: Press both dumbbells to extended position, bringing the dumbbells together over your chest. Slowly lower with control and repeat for the recommended repetitions.

Key Points: Maintain wrist position over the elbows. Do not allow your elbows to rotate inwards or outwards. Do not allow your head to jut forward.

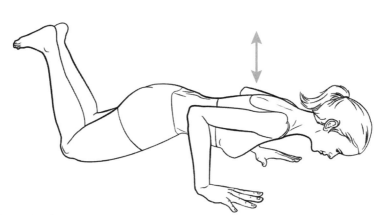

Kneeling Push-up

Starting Point: Place both hands on the floor in a kneeling position as shown. Activate your core.

Movement: While maintaining core stability, push up against the floor until both arms are fully extended. Slowly return until your body is just slightly above the floor. Repeat for the recommended repetitions.

Key Points: Maintain your core stability. Do not allow your head to jut forward. Do not lock your elbows on extension.

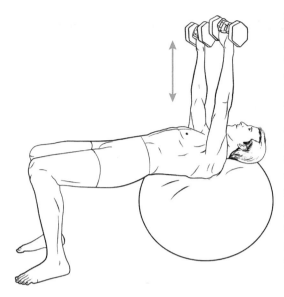

Dumbbell Chest Press

Starting Point: Lie on a ball with your head and shoulders positioned on the ball, a dumbbell in each hand. Your shoulders, hips, and knees should be aligned. Activate your core.

Movement: Press both dumbbells to an extended position, bringing the dumbbells together over your chest. Slowly lower with control and repeat for the recommended repetitions.

Key Points: Maintain wrist position over the elbows. Do not allow your elbows to rotate inwards or outwards. Do not allow your head to jut forward.

BACK STRENGTHENERS

One-Arm Dumbbell Row

Starting Point: Assume a 45-degree bent-over position with one arm extended, resting on a ball for support. Hold a dumbbell with your opposite arm hanging perpendicular to the floor. Activate your core.

Movement: While maintaining optimal posture, pull the dumbbell into the side of your chest. Slowly lower to the starting position and repeat for the recommended repetitions.

Key Points: Maintain your core stability. Focus on generating movement from your back, not your arms.

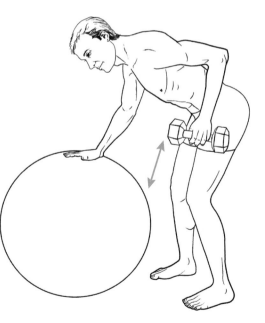

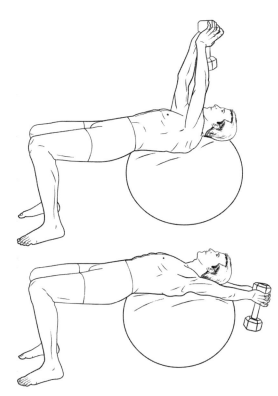

Dumbbell Pullover

Starting Point: Lie on a ball with your head and neck supported and with your hips aligned with your knees and shoulders. Hold one dumbbell in both hands over your chest. Activate your core.

Movement: While maintaining optimal posture, slowly lower the dumbbell backwards until the dumbbell is in line with your head. Using your back muscles, pull the dumbbell back to the starting position. Repeat for the recommended repetitions.

Key Points: Maintain your core stability and focus the movement through your back, not your arms. Keep both arms straight throughout the movement.

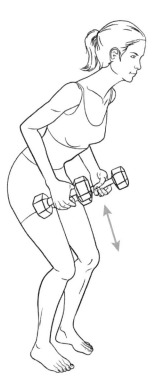

Dumbbell Row

Starting Point: Stand with your feet shoulder-width apart. Bend at your hip and knees. Hold a dumbbell in each hand with your palms facing your body. Assume a 45-degree bent-over position. Activate your core.

Movement: While maintaining optimal posture, pull the dumbbells in toward the side of your chest. Slowly lower to the starting position and repeat for the recommended repetitions.

Key Points: Maintain your core stability. Focus on generating movement from your back, not your arms.

SHOULDER STRENGTHENERS

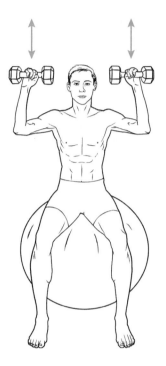

Dumbbell Shoulder Press (seated on ball)

Starting Point: Lie on a ball with your head and neck supported and with your hips aligned with your knees and shoulders. Hold one dumbbell in both hands over your chest. Activate your core.

Movement: While maintaining optimal posture, slowly lower the dumbbell backwards until the dumbbell is in line with your head. Using your back muscles, pull the dumbbell back to the starting position. Repeat for the recommended repetitions.

Key Points: Maintain your core stability and focus the movement through your back, not your arms. Keep both arms straight throughout the movement.

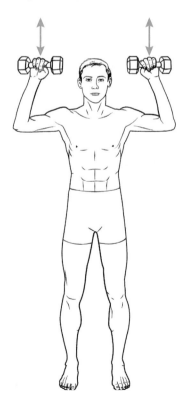

Dumbbell Shoulder Press

Starting Point: Stand with your feet shoulder-width apart. Bend at your hip and knees. Hold a dumbbell in each hand with your palms facing your body. Assume a 45-degree bent-over position. Activate your core.

Movement: While maintaining optimal posture, pull the dumbbells in toward the side of your chest. Slowly lower to the starting position and repeat for the recommended repetitions.

Key Points: Maintain your core stability. Focus on generating movement from your back, not your arms.

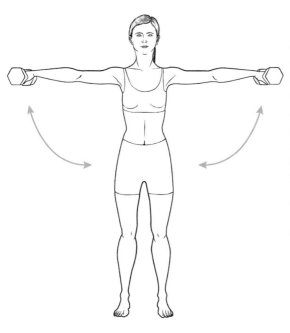

Dumbbell Lateral Raise

Starting Point: Stand with your feet shoulder-width apart, hips level, and toes pointing straight ahead. Hold a dumbbell in each hand at the sides. Activate your core.

Movement: While maintaining core activation, slowly raise both dumbbells laterally until they reach shoulder height. Slowly lower back to the starting position and repeat for the recommended repetitions.

Key Points: Maintain your core stability. Do not let your head jut forward. Look straight ahead.

BICEP STRENGTHENERS

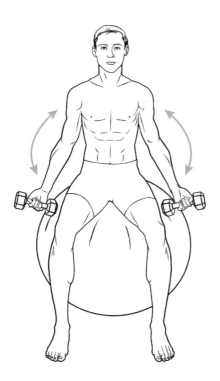

Dumbbell Curl (seated on ball)

Starting Point: Sit on a ball. Hold a dumbbell in each hand with your palms facing forward and arms extended. Activate your core.

Movement: Perform a dumbbell curl by flexing both elbows and raising the dumbbells toward your shoulders while keeping shoulder blades retracted. Slowly lower back to the original position by extending your elbows. Complete for the recommended repetitions.

Key Points: Maintain your core stability. Look straight ahead. Do not let your chin jut forward. Pivot from your elbows and keep them stationary.

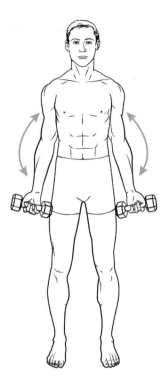

Standing Bicep Curl

Starting Point: Stand on both legs with feet pointing straight ahead and your knees slightly flexed. Hold one dumbbell each hand in, palms facing up with arms extended. Activate your core.

Movement: Perform a dumbbell curl by flexing both elbows and raising the dumbbells toward your shoulders while keeping the shoulder blades retracted. Slowly lower back to the original position by extending your elbows. Repeat for the recommended repetitions.

Key Points: Maintain your core stability. Look straight ahead. Do not let your chin jut forward. Pivot from your elbows and keep them stationary.

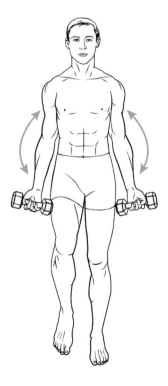

Standing Dumbbell Curl (on one leg)

Starting Point: Stand on one leg with the foot pointing straight ahead and knees slightly flexed. Hold one dumbbell in each hand, palms facing up with arms extended. Activate your core.

Movement: Perform a dumbbell curl by flexing both elbows and raising the dumbbells toward your shoulders while keeping the shoulder blades squeezed together. Slowly lower back to the original position by extending your elbows. Repeat for the recommended repetitions.

Key Points: Maintain your core stability. Look straight ahead. Do not let your chin jut forward. Pivot from your elbows and keep them stationary.

TRICEPS STRENGTHENERS

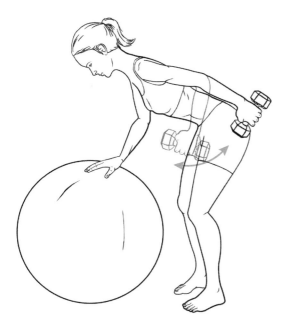

Dumbbell Kickback

Starting Point: Place exercise ball to the right of your body. While maintaining optimal alignment, lean forward from your hips and rest your right hand on the ball for support. Hold a dumbbell in the left hand. Activate your core.

Movement: Lift the upper left arm until it is parallel to the floor. While maintaining this upper arm position, slowly extend the elbow, hold, and return to the starting position. Repeat for the recommended repetitions and switch to the opposite arm.

Key Points: Maintain your core stability and keep your upper arm stationary and parallel to the floor. Do not hyper-extend the neck. Maintain a neutral head position.

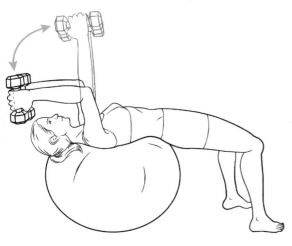

Lying Dumbbell Extension

Starting Point: Lie face up on a ball. Grip two dumbbells with both hands about12 inches apart. Activate your core.

Movement: Slowly lower the dumbbells to just slightly above your forehead. Extend both arms, returning to the starting position. Repeat for the recommended repetitions.

Key Points: Maintain your core activation. Keep the upper arms in a vertical position.

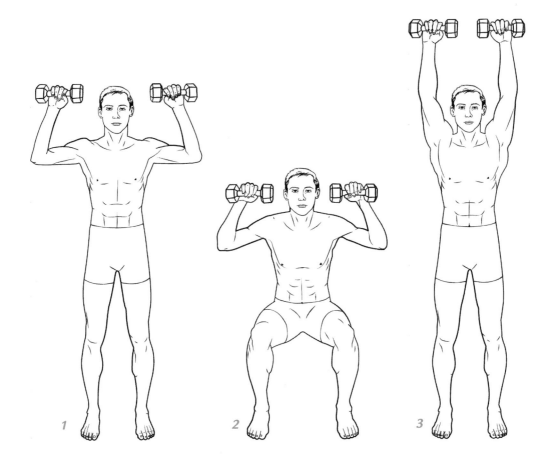

1   2   3

Squat and Press

Starting Point: Standing with a dumbbell in each hand and hands at shoulder level. Activate your core.

Movement: Squat until thighs are just past parallel to the floor. Extend both knees and hips and press both dumbbells over your head while returning to the starting position. Repeat for the recommended repetitions.

Key Points: Maintain your core activation. Do not let your chin jut forward. Maintain optimal posture while keeping both feet flat on the floor with equal weight distribution through your forefoot and heel.

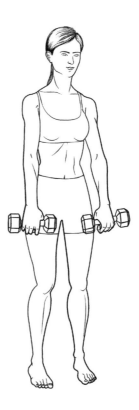

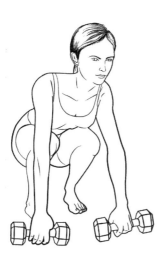

Dead Lift

Starting Point: Stand with your feet flat and shoulder-width apart. Squat and grasp a dumbbell in each hand with an overhand grip. Activate your core.

Movement: Lift both dumbbells from the ground by fully extending your hips and knees. Pull your shoulders back at the

top of the movement. Slowly return to the starting position and repeat for the recommended repetitions.

Key Points: Maintain your core activation. Keep the dumbbells close to your body with arms and back straight.

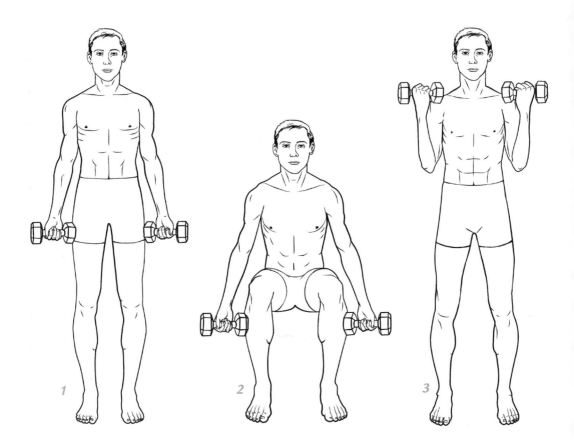

1 2 3

Dumbbell Squat with Bicep Curl

Starting Point: Stand with a dumbbell in each hand at your sides. Activate your core.

Movement: Descend until both thighs are just past parallel to the floor. Flex both elbows, curling the dumbbells to shoulder height while extending both of your knees and your hips to return to the starting position. Repeat for the recommended repetitions.

Key Points: Maintain your core activation. Do not let your chin jut forward. Maintain optimal posture while keeping both of your feet flat on the floor with equal weight distribution through forefoot and heel. Keep both elbows at your sides.

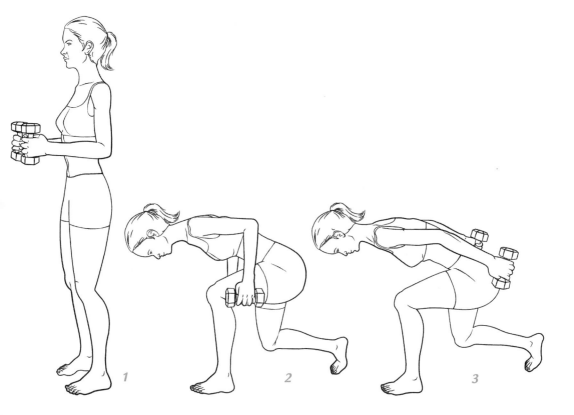

Forward Lunge with Triceps Extension

Starting Point: Stand with your feet shoulder-width apart. Bend both of your elbows to 90 degrees at your sides with a dumbbell in each hand. Activate your core.

Movement: Lunge forward with one leg, landing on your heel and then the forefoot. Lower your body by flexing the knee and hip of your forward leg until the knee of your rear leg is almost in contact with the floor. Bend at your waist until your torso is parallel to the ground. Extend both of your elbows, flexing the triceps. Return to the starting position by extending the knee and hip of your forward leg while bringing your torso upright and the dumbbells back to the starting position. Alternate your legs and repeat for the recommended repetitions.

Key Points: Maintain your core activation. Keep both elbows at your sides throughout the movement.

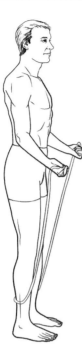

Skipping

Starting Point: Stand with both feet shoulder-width apart. Hold both handles of a skipping rope with your hands at your sides and the rope behind you. Activate your core.

Movement: Jump while simultaneously skipping over the rope. Continue skipping for the recommended time.

Key Points: Maintain your core activation while skipping.

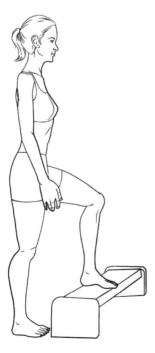

Step-ups

Starting Point: Stand with both hands at your sides and facing a bench or a step. Activate your core.

Movement: Place one foot on the bench. Step up on the bench. Return to the starting position by placing the foot of the first leg on the floor. Repeat stepping up and down on the bench as fast as possible while maintaining balance and control for the recommended time.

Key Points: Maintain your core activation. Keep your torso upright throughout the movement. Maintain balance. Be sure your whole foot makes contact with the bench.

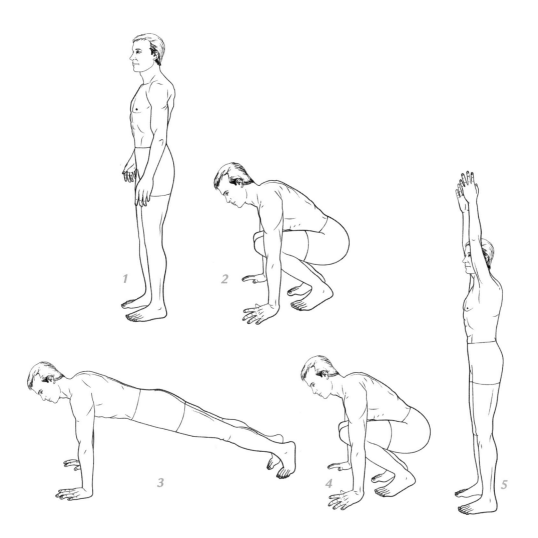

Burpees

Starting Point: Stand with both arms hanging at your sides. Position your feet about 12 inches apart. Activate your core.

Movement: Squat onto your hands and your toes. In a single motion, extend both of your legs back onto forefeet. Flex at the knees and hips, bringing both of your feet back under your shoulders and extend both knees and hips, returning to an upright position. Repeat for the recommended repetitions.

Key Points: Maintain your core activation. Keep your lower back flat—do not dip your hips toward the floor. Do not hyperextend your knees.

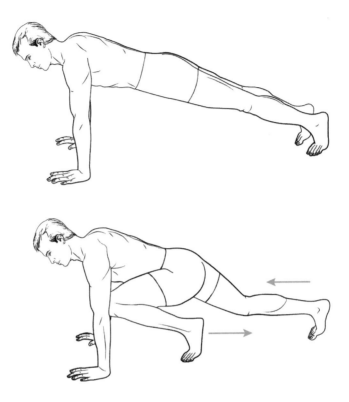

Mountain Climbers

Starting Point: Stand with both arms hanging at your sides. Position your feet about 12 inches apart. Activate your core.

Movement: Squat onto your hands and your toes. In a controlled motion, extend one leg back onto the forefoot. Flex at the knee and hip, bringing your foot back under your waist. Repeat for opposite leg.

Continue alternating, extending, and flexing each leg for the recommended amount of time.

Key Points: Maintain your core activation. Keep your lower back flat—do not let your hips dip toward the floor. Do not hyperextend your knees.

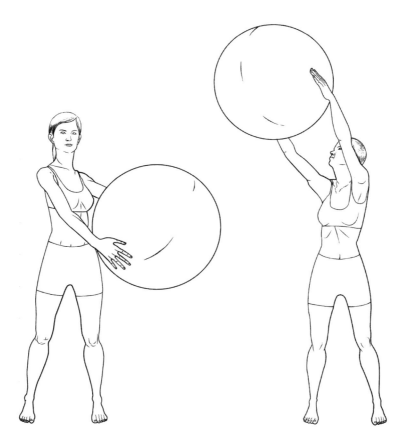

Reverse Wood Chops

Starting Point: Stand with your feet shoulder-width apart and feet pointing straight ahead with knees slightly flexed. Hold a ball in both hands at the outside of your left knee. Activate your core.

Movement: Extend both of your arms over the right shoulder in a reverse chopping motion. Slowly return to the starting position. Do the recommended repetitions and repeat with the opposite side.

Key Points: Maintain your core activation. Maintain proper arm position. Be sure to generate the movement from your trunk, not your arms.

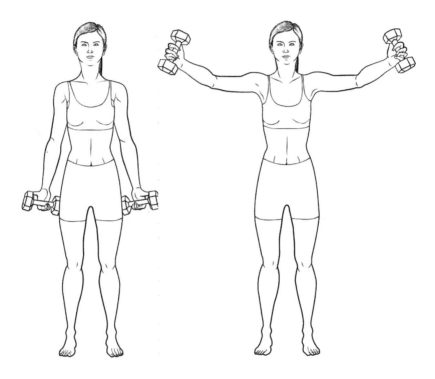

Standing Scaption

Starting Point: Stand with your feet shoulder-width apart, toes pointing straight ahead. Hold a dumbbell in each hand. Activate your core.

Movement: Raise both arms forward at a 45-degree angle while keeping one side of the dumbbell facing up. Raise it to your shoulder height only. Slowly lower to the starting position and repeat for the recommended repetitions.

Key Points: Maintain your core stability. Do not let your head jut forward. Look straight ahead.

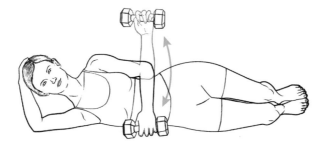

External Rotation

Starting Point: Lie on your right side on the floor, with your right hand supporting your head. Hold a dumbbell in the left hand. Activate your core.

Movement: While maintaining core stability and upper arm position, slowly externally rotate your left arm until your forearm is almost perpendicular to floor.

Slowly return to the starting position. Do the recommended repetitions and repeat with opposite side.

Key Points: Maintain your core stability. Keep your chest up and shoulders back. Maintain the correct arm position throughout the exercise.

PRE- AND POST-WORKOUT STRETCHES

Be sure to warm up for 10 minutes prior to stretching. A good warm-up consists of any low-impact rhythmic activity such as bike riding, walking, or using the elliptical machine. Hold each pre-workout stretch for 15–30 seconds and each post-workout stretch for 30–60 seconds. Breathe deeply and naturally, exhaling as you ease into each stretch. Do not bounce and be sure to ease slowly into and out of each stretch.

Right Neck Side Flexor Stretch

While maintaining good posture, hold down your right shoulder by tightening your back muscle. Tilt your head toward your left shoulder. Hold. Repeat three times and switch to the opposite side.

Lateral Shoulder Rotator Stretch

While maintaining good posture, reach behind your back with the right arm and grab hold of a towel or rope. The left arm should be overhead, pulling the towel/rope upward. Hold. Repeat three times and switch to the opposite side.

Right Chest Doorway Stretch

Standing close to a doorway, extend your right arm out to the side, parallel to the floor. Bend your elbow up, so that your palm faces forward in a "stop" position. Press your entire forearm and palm against the door jamb. Your upper arm should remain parallel to the floor. Keeping arm stationary, gently move your body into the doorway until you feel a stretch in your chest. Hold. Repeat three times and switch to the opposite side.

Kneeling Lat Stretch

Starting in a hands-and-knees position, raise your right arm and place it on a Swiss ball or chair with the palm facing up. Keeping the right arm extended, tuck in your pelvis. Slowly drop your body downward while keeping the pelvis position until you feel a stretch. Hold. Repeat the stretch three times and switch to the opposite side.

Triceps Stretch

While standing tall and maintaining good posture, raise your right arm overhead. Bend your elbow and place your right hand on your shoulder blade. Grab your elbow with your left hand and push back. Hold. Repeat three times and switch to the opposite side.

Right Gluteus Maximus and External Hip Rotator Stretch

Lie on your back and cross your right leg over your left knee. Bring your left knee forward toward your chest. Keep your head, shoulders, and back flat on the floor. Continue until you feel the stretch in the gluteus and hip muscles. Hold. Repeat three times and switch to the opposite side.

Lying Hip Flexor Stretch

While lying on your left side, flex your left hip and pull your thigh close to your chest. Use your hand for stabilization, and tuck in your pelvis. Straighten your right leg. Bend your knee, grasp your ankle, and pull your heel toward your buttock. Hold for 20 seconds. Repeat three times and switch to the opposite side.

Kneeling Lunge Stretch

Start in a lunge position, right leg forward, left knee on the ground, and tuck in your pelvis. Slowly move your body forward until you feel a stretch in the front of the left hip. Hold. Repeat three times and switch to the opposite side.

Lying Lower Hamstring Stretch

While lying on your back, bend your right hip and knee to 90 degrees. Do not arch your back. Keep your lower back neutral. Instead of pointing your toes away from you, flex your toes. Slowly straighten your leg by extending your knee toward the ceiling until you feel a stretch. Your thigh must not move. Hold. Repeat three times and switch to the opposite side.

Gastrocnemius Stretch

While standing near and facing a wall, bring your left leg forward and lean your upper body forward, placing both hands on the wall. Your back leg should remain straight and your rear foot should remain flat with toes pointed straight ahead. Bend both arms, and move your upper body further toward the wall. Continue until you feel a stretch. Hold. Repeat three times and switch to the opposite side.

Soleus Stretch

While standing near and facing a wall, bring your left leg forward and lean your upper body forward, placing both hands on the wall. Your back leg should remain straight and your rear foot should remain flat with toes pointed straight ahead. Bend your rear knee until you feel a stretch. Hold. Repeat three times and switch to the opposite side.

ACTION
Perform the preceding pre- and post-workout stretches each time that you perform a resistance-training workout.

THE WORKOUTS

17

This chapter contains the workouts you are to follow on the Fat-Fighter Diet program. For those of you who work out at the gym, at the end of this chapter I have included a blank workout sheet for you to copy, fill, and take with you.

Begin each workout by completing a light five-minute cardiovascular warm-up followed immediately by the pre-workout stretch routine on pages 183–85. Next, simply choose the workout level and stream that are right for you. After finishing your resistance training, cool down by performing your post-workout stretches.

Please pay careful attention to the intensity, tempo, and rest interval suggestions and always use proper form. Never sacrifice form for an increase in weight. Most importantly, have fun and enjoy yourself! This is your body and each workout is going to make you stronger, leaner, and healthier.

Definition of Fitness Training Terms

Throughout the proceeding workouts you will see many terms that may not be familiar to you. Please refer to the following list of explanations for each training term.

Circuit: A series of three or more exercises performed consecutively with no rest in between.

Drop set: A set of an exercise that decreases in weight and increases in repetitions. There is no rest between each weight change of the set. For example, if under "Rep" it says 6–8–15, first complete 6 reps, then decrease weight and complete 8 reps, and finish by decreasing weight once more and complete 15 reps. Repeat as recommended.

Intensity: A percentage of your maximum ability for a given exercise, with 100 percent intensity meaning you could do only one rep of that exercise (1RM [1 rep max] = 100 percent intensity, 5RM = 50 percent intensity).

Rest interval: The amount of rest taken in between sets of an exercise(s).

Superset: Two exercises performed back to back with no rest in between.

Tempo: The speed of each repetition. The first digit is the lowering (negative) portion, the middle digit is the pause, and the third digit is the return (positive) movement. An asterisk (*) is used to denote "as fast as possible." This can be illustrated by looking at a bicep curl with a tempo of 3/1/1. Starting with elbows flexed, lower the dumbbells for three seconds, pause at the bottom for one second, and then take another second to return the dumbbells to the shoulder level starting position.

THE FAT LOSS STREAM

Fat Loss: Beginner

Perform the following workout on three nonconsecutive days per week (e.g., M/W/S). Repeat for four weeks and proceed to Intermediate Phase 1.

Body Part	Exercises	Work Sets	Rep	Intensity	Tempo	Rest Interval (sec)
Core	Pelvic tilt	1–2	5	Bodyweight	5/0/5	60
Core	Side plank (on knees)	1–2	n/a	Bodyweight	30–60 sec	60
Core	Front plank (on knees)	1–2	n/a	Bodyweight	30–60 sec	60
Quads	Ball squat	1–2	12–15	Bodyweight	3/1/1	60
Core	Quadruped (on floor)	1–2	1–8 per side	Bodyweight	5/1/5	60
Chest	Kneeling push-up	1–2	12–15	Bodyweight	3/1/1	60
Back	One arm dumbbell row	1–2	12–15	65–70%	3/1/1	60
Back	Dumbbell pullover (on ball)	1–2	12–15	65–70%	3/1/1	60
Shoulders	Dumbbell shoulder press (seated on ball)	1–2	12–15	65–70%	3/1/1	60
Biceps	Dumbbell curl (seated on ball)	1–2	12–15	65–70%	3/1/1	60
Triceps	Dumbbell triceps (kickback)	1–2	12–15	65–70%	3/1/1	60
Abdominal	Crunch (on ball)	1–2	12–15	Bodyweight	3/3/3	60

Fat Loss: Intermediate

Perform the following workout on three nonconsecutive days per week (e.g., M/W/S). Repeat for four weeks and proceed to Advanced Phase 1.

| Body Part | Exercises | Warm-up | | Work | | Intensity | Tempo | Rest Interval |
		Sets	Rep	Sets	Rep			
Core	Front plank on toes	1	n/a	2	n/a	Bodyweight	30–60 sec	start superset
Core	Side plank (on knees)	1	n/a	2	n/a	Bodyweight	30–60 sec	end superset
Quads	Dumbbell squat	1	12	2	10–12	70–75%	3/1/1	start superset
Back	Dumbbell row (standing)	1	12	2	10–12	70–75%	3/1/1	end superset
Abs (upper)	Crunch (on ball)	1	12	2	10	Bodyweight	3/1/3	start superset
Chest	Dumbbell chest press (on ball)	1	12	2	10–12	70–75%	3/1/1	end superset
Quads	Front lunge	1	12	2	10–12	70–75%	3/1/1	start superset
Back	One-arm dumbbell row (on ball)	1	12	2	10–12	70–75%	3/1/1	end superset
Abs (upper)	Crunch (on ball)	1	12	2	10	Bodyweight	3/1/3	start superset
Shoulders	Dumbbell shoulder press (on ball)	1	12	2	10–12	70–75%	3/1/1	end superset
Abs (lower)	Reverse crunch (on floor)	1	12	1	10	Bodyweight	3/1/3	start superset
Biceps	Dumbbell curl (on ball)	1	12	1	10–12	70–75%	3/1/1	end superset
Abs (lower)	Knees up (supine)	1	12	1	10	Bodyweight	3/1/3	start superset
Triceps	Lying dumbbell triceps extension (on ball)	1	12	1	10–12	70–75%	3/1/1	end superset

Fat Loss: Advanced

Perform the following workout for four weeks on three nonconsecutive days per week (e.g., M/W/S).

Body Part	Exercises	Warm-up Sets	Warm-up Rep	Work Sets	Work Rep	Intensity	Tempo	Rest Interval
Total body	Squat and press (dumbbell)	1	10	2	6–8	75–85%	1/0/*	start circuit
Chest	Incline press (on ball)	1	10	2	6–8	75–85%	2/1/1	
Active rest	Skipping	–	–	2	n/a	Bodyweight	1 min	end circuit
Quads	Dumbbell squat	1	10	2	6–8	75–85%	2/1/1	start circuit
Back	Dumbbell pullover (on ball)	1	10	2	6–8	75–85%	2/1/1	
Active rest	Step-ups	–	–	2	n/a	Bodyweight	1 min	end circuit
Total body	Dead lift dumbbell	1	10	2	6–8	75–85%	2/1/1	start circuit
Shoulders	Dumbbell shoulder press (standing)	1	10	2	6–8	75–85%	2/1/1	
Active rest	Burpees	–	–	2	n/a	Bodyweight	1 min	end circuit
Total body	Dumbbell squat with bicep curl	1	12	2	8–10	75–85%	2/1/1	start circuit
Abs (upper)	Crunch (on ball)	1	12	2	10	70–75%	3/1/1	
Active Rest	Mountain climbers	–	–	2	n/a	Bodyweight	1 min	end circuit
Total body	Forward lunge with triceps extension	1	12	2	8–10	75–85%	2/1/1	start circuit
Abs (lower)	Reverse crunch	1	12	2	10	Bodyweight	3/1/1	
Active rest	Skipping	–	–	2	n/a	Bodyweight	1 min	end circuit
Total body	Wood chops with medicine ball	1	12	2	8–10	75–80%	1/0/*	start circuit
Core	Side plank (on toes)	1	n/a	2	n/a	Bodyweight	30–60 sec	
Active rest	Step-ups	–	–	2	n/a	Bodyweight	1 min	end circuit

THE HEALTHY LIFESTYLE STREAM

Healthy Lifestyle: Beginner

Perform the following workout on three nonconsecutive days per week (e.g., M/W/S). Repeat for four weeks and proceed to Intermediate Phase 1.

Body Part	Exercises	Work		Intensity	Tempo	Rest Interval (sec)
		Sets	Rep			
Core	Pelvic tilt	1–2	5	Bodyweight	5/0/5	60
Core	Side plank (on knees)	1–2	5	Bodyweight	30–60 sec	60
Core	Front plank (on knees)	1–2	n/a	Bodyweight	30–60 sec	60
Quads	Ball squat	1–2	12–15	Bodyweight	3/1/1	60
Core	Quadruped (on floor)	1–2	8 per side	Bodyweight	5/1/5	60
Chest	Kneeling push-up	1–2	12–15	Bodyweight	3/1/1	60
Back	One-arm dumbbell row	1–2	12–15	65–70%	3/1/1	60
Back	Dumbbell pullover (on ball)	1–2	12–15	65–70%	3/1/1	60
Shoulders	Dumbbell shoulder press (seated on ball)	1–2	12–15	65–70%	3/1/1	60
Biceps	Dumbbell curl (seated on ball)	1–2	12–15	65–70%	3/1/1	60
Triceps	Dumbbell triceps (kickback)	1–2	12–15	65–70%	3/1/1	60
Abdominal	Crunch (on ball)	1–2	12–15	Bodyweight	3/3/3	60

Healthy Lifestyle: Intermediate

In this phase, you will increase the weight you lift. Perform this workout on three nonconsecutive days per week (e.g., M/W/S). Repeat for four weeks and proceed to Advanced Phase 1.

Body Part	Exercises	Warm-up		Work		Intensity	Tempo	Rest Interval (sec)
		Sets	Rep	Sets	Rep			
Abs (lower)	Knees up (supine)	1	12	2	10	Bodyweight	3/1/1	60
Core	Front plank (on toes)	1	12	2	n/a	Bodyweight	30–60 sec	60
Abs (upper)	Crunch (on ball)	1	12	2	15–20	Bodyweight	3/1/3	60
Quads	Dumbbell squat	1	12	2	10–12	70–75%	3/1/1	60
Chest	Dumbbell chest press (on ball)	1	12	2	10–12	70–75%	3/1/1	60
Back	One-arm dumbbell row (on ball)	1	12	2	10–12	70–75%	3/1/1	60
Back 2	Dumbbell pullover (on ball)	1	12	2	10–12	70–75%	3/1/1	60
Shoulders	Dumbbell shoulder press (standing)	1	12	2	10–12	70–75%	3/1/1	60
Biceps	Standing dumbbell curl	1	12	2	10–12	70–75%	3/1/1	60
Triceps	Lying dumbbell triceps extension (on ball)	1	12	2	10–12	70–75%	3/1/1	60
Lower back	Quadruped (on knees)	1	12	2	10	Bodyweight	3/3/3	60

Healthy Lifestyle: Advanced

In this phase you will increase the amount you will lift again. Perform this workout for four weeks on three nonconsecutive days per week (e.g., M/W/S).

Body Part	Exercises	Warm-up Sets	Warm-up Rep	Work Sets	Work Rep	Intensity	Tempo	Rest Interval
Total body	Squat and press (dumbbell)	1	10	2	6–8	75–85%	1/0	2 min
Quads	Dumbbell squat	1	10	2	6–8	75–85%	2/1/1	2 min
Chest	Dumbbell chest press (on ball)	1	10	2	6–8	75–85%	2/1/1	60 sec
Back	One-arm dumbbell row (on ball)	1	10	2	6–8	75–85%	2/1/1	2 min
Biceps	Dumbbell curl (standing on one leg)	1	10	2	10	70–75%	3/1/1	1 min
Triceps	Lying dumbbell triceps extension (on ball)	1	10	2	10	70–75%	3/1/1	1 min
Core	Front plank	–	–	2	n/a	Bodyweight	30–60 sec	60 sec
Core	Side plank (on toes)	–	–	2	n/a	Bodyweight	30–60 sec	60 sec

THE INCREASE LEAN MUSCLE AND STRENGTH STREAM

Increase Muscle: Beginner

Perform the following workout on three nonconsecutive days per week (e.g., M/W/S). Repeat for four weeks and proceed to Intermediate Phase 1.

Body Part	Exercises	Work Sets	Rep	Intensity	Tempo	Rest Interval (sec)
Core	Pelvic tilt	1-2	5	Bodyweight	5/0/5	60
Core	Bridge (on floor)	1-2	5	Bodyweight	30/5/0	60
Core	Front plank (on knees)	1-2	n/a	Bodyweight	30-60 sec	60
Quads	Ball squat	1-2	12-15	Bodyweight	2/1/1	60
Core	Quadruped (on floor)	1-2	8 per side	Bodyweight	5/1/5	60
Chest	Kneeling push-up	1-2	12-15	Bodyweight	3/1/1	60
Back	One-arm dumbbell row	1-2	12-15	65-70%	3/1/1	60
Back	Dumbbell Pullover (on ball)	1-2	12-15	65-70%	3/1/1	60
Shoulders	Dumbbell shoulder press (seated on ball)	1-2	12-15	65-70%	3/1/1	60
Biceps	Dumbbell curl (seated on ball)	1-2	12-15	65-70%	3/1/1	60
Triceps	Dumbbell triceps (kickback)	1-2	12-15	65-70%	3/1/1	60
Abdominal	Crunch (on ball)	1-2	12-15	Bodyweight	3/3/3	60

Increase Muscle: Intermediate

Perform the following workout on three nonconsecutive days per week (e.g., M/W/S). Repeat for four weeks and proceed to Advanced Phase 1.

Body Part	Exercises	Warm-up		Work		Intensity	Tempo	Rest Interval
		Sets	Rep	Sets	Rep			
Abs (lower)	Knees up (supine)	1	12	2	10	Bodyweight	3/1/3	start circuit
Core	Side plank (on toes)	1	n/a	2	n/a	Bodyweight	30–60 sec	
Abs	Russian twist	1	12	2	10	Bodyweight	3/1/3	end circuit
Back	Standing scaption	1	15	–	–	55–65%	3/1/3	start superset
Rotator cuff	External rotation	1	15	–	–	55–65%	3/1/3	end superset
Quads	Dumbbell squat	1	12	2	6–8	75–85%	3/1/1	start superset
Hamstring	Hamstring curl (on ball)	1	12	2	6–8	Ball	3/1/1	end superset
Back	One-arm dumbbell row (on ball)	1	12	2	6–8	75–85%	2/1/1	start superset
Chest	Incline dumbbell press (on ball)	1	12	2	6–8	75–85%	2/1/1	end superset
Shoulders	Dumbbell shoulder press (seated)	1	12	1–2	6/8/15	65–85%	2/1/1	drop set
Biceps	Standing bicep curl	1	12	1–2	12–15	60–75%	2/1/1	start superset
Triceps	Lying triceps extension (ball)	1	12	1–2	12–15	60–75%	2/1/1	end superset

Increase Muscle: Advanced

Perform the following workout for four weeks on three nonconsecutive days per week (e.g., M/W/S).

Body Part	Exercises	Warm-up Sets	Warm-up Rep	Work Sets	Work Rep	Intensity	Tempo	Rest Interval
Abs (lower)	Crunch (on ball)	1	12	2	10	Bodyweight	3/1/3	start circuit
Core	Knees up (supine)	1	n/a	2	n/a	Bodyweight	30–60 sec	
Core	Side plank (on toes)	1	12	2	10	Bodyweight	3/2/1	end circuit
Back	Standing scaption	1	15	–	–	55–65%	3/1/3	start superset
Rotator cuff	External rotation	1	15	–	–	55–65%	3/1/3	end superset
Quads	Dumbbell squat	1	12	3	8/12/20	75–85%	3/1/1	2 dropset
Chest	Dumbbell chest press (on ball)	1	12	3	6–8	75–85%	3/1/1	start superset
Back	Dumbbell row (standing)	1	12	3	6–8	75–85%	2/1/1	end superset
Shoulders	Dumbbell lateral raise (standing)	1	12	2	8–12	75–85%	2/1/1	start superset
Shoulders	Dumbbell shoulder press (seated)	1	12	2	8–12	75–85%	2/1/1	end superset
Triceps	Lying triceps extension (on ball)	1	12	1–2	6/8/15	65–85%	2/1/1	drop set
Biceps	Standing bicep curl	1	12	1–2	6/8/15	65–85%	2/1/1	drop set

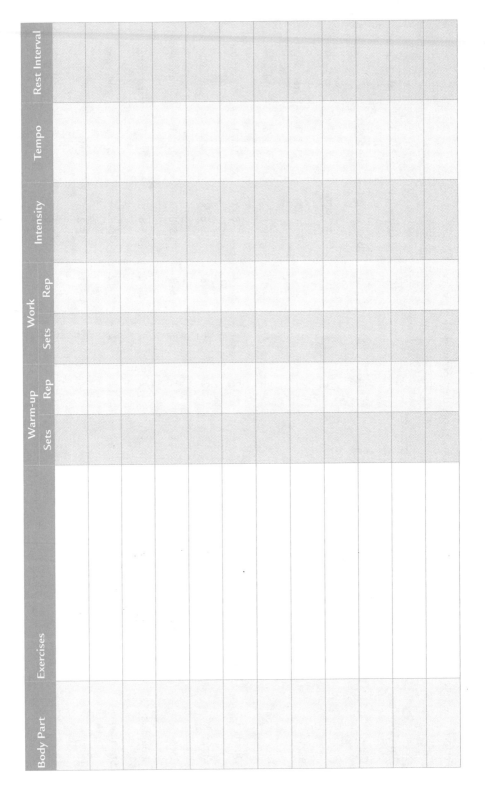

| Body Part | Exercises | Warm-up | | Work | | Intensity | Tempo | Rest Interval |
		Sets	Rep	Sets	Rep			

I DID IT! NOW WHAT?

Most of us will spend days, weeks, months, or even years lamenting over a failure, but we rarely remember to take the time to celebrate a moment of success. This is a mistake! For every goal (both small and large) that you achieve, be sure to do three very important things: Reward, remind, and reinvest!

1. REWARD YOURSELF

We all respond favorably to positive reinforcement. It is a scientific fact that what gets rewarded gets repeated. The rule of consequence simply states that consequences (such as having a nice meal at your favorite restaurant, taking a day-trip to a favorite place, or receiving a relaxing massage) will increase behavior (such as exercising five or six days per week, eating five small meals per day, or remembering to take your supplements all week).

This rule provides an excellent blueprint for influence. If you want to increase a behavior, then provide a consequence of reward when the behavior is shown. For every goal that you achieve, be sure to reward yourself with something positive that will increase the behavior. Though your new level of energy and active, healthy body may seem like reward enough, don't be stingy with yourself! You deserve wonderful rewards for all your hard work and dedication.

2. REMIND YOURSELF

Nothing succeeds like success. Begin a collection of motivational and inspirational e-mails, articles, videos, and before and after pictures of yourself.

Positive reminders are important in producing changes in physical activity and nutrition-related behavior. Any time you feel demotivated or that you can't carry on with the program, simply go back and review your collection of motivational and inspirational materials. This will remind you that you, in fact, *can* do it!

3. REINVEST YOURSELF

Don't stop now! Be sure to set *new* goals. Setting goals is the secret to staying motivated and will fill you with the purpose and enthusiasm to keep you moving forward. After each achievement, set new behavior and outcome goals. Establish new reasons for achieving these goals and set deadlines for their accomplishment. Build on your success and strive to go to the next level. Goal setting should never stop. You will always have a feeling of purpose when you are working on achieving something you strongly desire. This purposeful life will be filled with energy and enthusiasm as long as you are moving toward the achievement of a goal. You are the author of your own destiny—design the life of your dreams.

ACTION

Always be sure to reward yourself for a job well done. Positively reinforce your new mindset, behaviors, and achievements. Set new goals that excite and inspire you. Goal setting never stops!

TRANSFORM WORDS INTO ACTION!

To Do List:
- Get beyond your exercise myths.
- Perform the correct amount of cardio for your goal.
- Determine and perform the correct resistance-training workout for you.
- Stretch before and after each workout.
- Reward yourself for your accomplishments.

As you can see, exercise is an essential component to achieving your Fat Fighter goals. I hope that this book has infused into your consciousness the importance of exercising when you are setting out to improve your health and lose body fat. I trust that you now understand why resistance training, in particular, is vital to changing your body composition and tipping the scales from fat to lean.

In addition, you understand how a periodized training program works; the importance of including resistance, strength, and cardio training as part of an effective workout routine; and how to tailor your workout to suit your goal. For optimal results, perform cardio exercise on alternate days while keeping each workout to less than 45 minutes. This combination of periodized resistance training, together with cardiovascular conditioning and stretching, is guaranteed to yield terrific results for years to come.

OVERVIEW

Knowing is not enough, you must apply; willing is not enough, you must do.

—Bruce Lee

Congratulations! You now know more about health, fitness, and fat loss than 90 percent of the population (or more). You're an expert! However, please do not become one of the millions who simply read and never apply. It is only through the application of this knowledge that you will begin to see results.

You have made it to the end of this book, not your journey. Your journey to a life filled with hope, fitness, vibrant energy, and health in a lean and strong body is just beginning. I encourage you to find a friend to join you on this journey. Support and encourage one another. Remember that success shared is twice as sweet, plus it has 0 calories and absolutely no impact on blood sugar!

Enjoy this journey! Find the pleasure that is in the process of becoming successful—you will never regret it.

PRODUCT RESOURCES

Omega-3 Fish Oil Suggestions
- Omega-3 extra strength from Genuine Health
- Super Omega-3 EPA/DHA from Life Extension
- EPA-DHA Balanced Liquid from Metagenics

Green Drink Suggestions
- Greens+ from Genuine Health
- Life Extension Herbal Mix from Life Extension

Multivitamin and Mineral Suggestions
- Multi+ complete or greens+multi+ from Genuine Health
- Life Extension Mix
- Multigenics from Metagenics

CLA Suggestions
- Abs+ from Genuine Health
- Super CLA Blend from Life Extension
- Ultra CLA from Metagenics

Green Tea Suggestions
- Any organic green tea blend of your choice

HCA Suggestions

· Leans+ from Genuine Health
· HCA from Life Extension

Fiber Suggestions

· Satisfiber+ from Genuine Health
· Enhanced Fiber Food Powder from Life Extension
· MetaFiber from Metagenics

Whey Proteins Suggestions

· Proteins+ from Genuine Health
· Enhanced Life Extension Protein
· Perfect Protein from Metagenics

Creatine Suggestions

· Micronized Creatine from Life Extension

R-Alpha Lipoic Acid Suggestions

· Super Alpha Lipoic Acid from Life Extension

BIBLIOGRAPHY

The following references were reviewed to help develop *The Fat-Fighter Diet*.

Aceto, C. *Everything you need to know about fat loss.* Lewiston, Maine: Club Creavalle, Inc. 1997.

Black, H.R. "The coronary artery disease paradox: The role of hyperinsulinemia and insulin resistance and implications for therapy." *Journal of Cardiovascular Pharmacology.* 15 (1990) S26–S38.

Colgan, M. *Optimum Sports Nutrition.* New York: Advanced Research Press, 1993.

Faigin, R. *Natural Hormone Enhancement.* Cedar Mountain, NC: Extique Publishing, 2000.

Frayn, K.N., et al. "Coordinated regulation of hormone-sensitive lipase and lipoprotein lipase in human adipose tissue in vivo: Implications for the control of fat storage and fat mobilization." *Advances in Enzyme Regulation.* 35 (1995) 163–178.

Goldfine, I.D. "Effects of insulin on intracellular processes." *Biochem Action Hormones.* 8 (1981) 273–305.

Graci, S. *The Bone-Building Solution*. Toronto: John Wiley and Sons Canada, 2006.

Graci, S. *The Path to Phenomenal Health*. Toronto: John Wiley and Sons Canada, 2005.

Graci, S. *The Food Connection*. Toronto: Macmillan Canada, 2001.

Grundy, S.M., MD, Phd., et al. "Comparison of monounsaturated fatty acids and carbohydrates for reducing raised levels of plasma cholesterol in man." *American Journal of Clinical Nutrition*. 47 (1988) 965–969.

Hales, C.N., Luzio, J.P., and Liddle, K. "Hormonal control of adipose tissue lipolysis." *Biochemical Society Symposia*. 43 (1978) 97–135.

Hickson, J.F., and Wolinski, I., Eds. *Nutrition in Exercise and Sport, 2nd edition*. Boca Raton, FL: CRC Press, 1994.

Hill, N. *Think and Grow Rich*. City: Penguin Group, 2003.

Ivy, J., and Portman, R. *Nutrient Timing*. Laguna Beach, CA: Basic Health Publications, 2004.

Katan, M.B., Zock, P.L., and Mensink, R.P. "Dietary oils, serum lipoproteins, and coronary heart disease." *American Journal of Clinical Nutrition*. 61(suppl) (1995) 1368S–1373S.

Keins, B., et al. "Lipoprotein lipase activity and intramuscular triglycerides stores after long-term high fat and high carbohydrate diets in physically trained men." *Clinical Physiology*. 7 (1987) 1–9.

Kraemer, W.J. *Strength and Power in Sport*. Ed. by Komi, P. Oxford: Blackwell Scientific, 1992.

McCargar, L.J., Baracoc, V.E., and Clandinin, M.T. "Influence of dietary carbohydrate-to-fat ratio on whole body nitrogen retention and body composition in adult rats." *Journal of Nurtition*. 119 (1989) 1240–1245.

McCargar L.J., et al. "Dietary carbohydrate-to-fat ratio: Influence on whole body nitrogen retention, substrate utilization, and hormone response in healthy male subjects." *American Journal of Clinical Nutrition*. 49 (1989) 1169–1178.

Merrill, A.H. *"Lipid modulators of cell function."* *Nutrition Reviews*. 47 (6) (1989) 161–169.

Muller, W.A., et al "The influence of the antecedent diet upon glucagons and insulin secretio.", *New England Journal of Medicine*. 285 (1971) 1450-1454.

Poliquin, C. *The Poliquin Principles*. Napa: Dayton Publication and Writers Group, 1997

Schwarzenegger, A. *Encyclopedia of Modern Bodybuilding*. New York: Simon and Schuster, 1985.

Roth, J., et al. "The influence of blood glucose on the plasma concentration of growth hormone." *Diabetes*. 13 (1964) 355–361.

Sebokova, E., et al. "Alteration of the lipid composition of rat testicular plasma membranes by dietary fatty acids changes the responsiveness of leydig cells and testosterone synthesis." *Journal of Nutrition*. 120 (1990) 160–168.

Swislocki, A.M., et al. "Insulin suppression of plasma free fatty acid concentration in normal individuals or patients with Type 2 diabetes." *Diabetologia*. 30 (1987) 622.

Pharmacology. 15 (1990) S26–S38.

Unger, R.H., MD. "Glucagon and the insulin: Glucagon ratio in diabetes and other catabolic illnesses." *Diabetes*. 20 (December 1971)(12) 834–838.

INDEX

Body Part	Exercises	Warm-up		Work		Intensity	Tempo	Rest Interval
		Sets	Rep	Sets	Rep			

| Body Part | Exercises | Warm-up | | Work | | | Intensity | Tempo | Rest Interval |
		Sets	Rep	Sets	Rep				

| Body Part | Exercises | Warm-up | | Work | | | Intensity | Tempo | Rest Interval |
		Sets	Rep	Sets	Rep				

Body Part	Exercises	Warm-up		Work		Intensity	Tempo	Rest Interval
		Sets	Rep	Sets	Rep			

Body Part	Exercises	Warm-up		Work		Intensity	Tempo	Rest Interval
		Sets	Rep	Sets	Rep			

| Body Part | Exercises | Warm-up | | Work | | Intensity | Tempo | Rest Interval |
		Sets	Rep	Sets	Rep			

Body Part	Exercises	Warm-up		Work		Intensity	Tempo	Rest Interval
		Sets	Rep	Sets	Rep			

FOLLOW THE FAT-FIGHTER DIET ONLINE!

You have read the book, now get with the program!

You can have your own Fat-Fighter nutrition and exercise program created for you for a fraction of what it would cost to train one on one with Bruce.

With thousands of meal plans, recipes, workout routines, and exercise videos, eBodi.com is the world's most comprehensive, healthy, fat-loss resource.

Visit www.fatfighterdiet.com or www.ebodi.com for your personalized program today!

ENERGIZE YOUR COMPANY!

Bruce Krahn, author of *The Fat-Fighter Diet* and president of eBodi.com will speak to your team live!

Add life, energy, health, and inspiration to your next conference or meeting.

Also available—Live Lean at Lunch. These Lunch & Learn sessions are perfect for companies of all sizes.

Contact us at speakers@ebodi.com for more information.